Returning to the Source

of related interest

The Art and Practice of Diagnosis in Chinese Medicine
Nigel Ching
Foreword by Jeremy Halpin
ISBN 978 1 84819 314 7
eISBN 978 0 85701 267 8

Kampo
A Clinical Guide to Theory and Practice, Second Edition
Keisetsu Otsuka
Foreword by Dan Bensky
ISBN 978 1 84819 329 1
eISBN 978 0 85701 286 9

The Fundamentals of Acupuncture
Nigel Ching
Foreword by Charles Buck
ISBN 978 1 84819 313 0
eISBN 978 0 85701 266 1

The Yellow Monkey Emperor's Classic of Chinese Medicine
Damo Mitchell and Spencer Hill
Illustrated by Spencer Hill
ISBN 978 1 84819 286 7
eISBN 978 0 85701 233 3

The Essential Teachings of Sasang Medicine
An Annotated Translation of Lee Je-ma's Dongeui Susei Bowon
Gary Wagman
ISBN 978 1 84819 317 8
eISBN 978 0 85701 270 8

RETURNING TO THE SOURCE

Han Dynasty Medical Classics in Clinical Practice

Z'ev Rosenberg

Edited and with contributions by DANIEL SCHRIER
Foreword by SABINE WILMS
Afterword by KEN ROSE

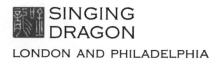

SINGING
DRAGON

LONDON AND PHILADELPHIA

First published in 2018
by Singing Dragon
an imprint of Jessica Kingsley Publishers
73 Collier Street
London N1 9BE, UK
and
400 Market Street, Suite 400
Philadelphia, PA 19106, USA

www.singingdragon.com

Library of Congress Cataloging in Publication Data
Names: Rosenberg, Z'ev, LAc, author.
Title: Returning to the source : Han Dynasty medical classics in clinical
    practice / Z'ev Rosenberg.
Description: London ; Philadelphia : Jessica Kingsley Publishers, 2018. |
    Includes bibliographical references.
Identifiers: LCCN 2017044159| ISBN 9781848193482 (alk. paper) | ISBN
    9780857013064 (eISBN)
Subjects: | MESH: Medicine, Chinese Traditional--methods | Philosophy, Medical
Classification: LCC R601 | NLM WB 55.C4 | DDC 610.951--dc23
LC record available at https://lccn.loc.gov/2017044159

British Library Cataloguing in Publication Data
A CIP catalogue record for this book is available from the British Library

ISBN 978 1 84819 348 2
eISBN 978 0 85701 306 4

Printed and bound in Great Britain

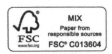

*Dedicated to my mother, Jacqueline, who
lived 95 healthy and happy years, and
Rabbi Meir Michel Abehsera, who taught me
how to 'return to the source' in so many ways...*

Contents

Praise for Returning to the Source

Dr. Z'ev Rosenberg has been practicing East Asian medicine for over 30 years. For all intents and purposes, and especially by Chinese standards, this makes him one of the first non-Chinese *minglao zhongyi* 名老中醫, or 'famous old Chinese physicians' in the Occident. But this is hardly a qualifying factor for Z'ev's success and wide acclaim as an educator and clinician.

Through these past four decades, Z'ev has been an ardent proponent of the renaissance of the classical style of Chinese medicine practice, regardless of the ever-increasing onslaught of contemporary trends and calls for the modernization of Chinese medicine. For decades, even when translations of many classical writings were scarcely available, Z'ev has been hard at work not only championing the classics, but also trying to elucidate their deeper meaning, and integrate their wisdom into the practical application in daily clinical routine. This is Dr. Rosenberg's greatest asset and contribution to the field.

And so it is no surprise that, in the autumn of a very successful life of living the ancient way, in word and deed, Z'ev has finally decided to share with us his unique insights and understanding of Chinese medicine, as cultivated throughout his academic and professional life. Not only does he share his specific perspectives and approaches to the classical knowledge, he also argues to teach from the classics, and not merely about the classics. His successful professional career is testament to the viability of this conviction.

In this current day and age where true Chinese medicine has virtually been severed at the root, this book is an invaluable encouragement to budding practitioners and seasoned experts alike, demonstrating that the only way to master the medicine and impart a lasting beneficial effect on one's patients, is to commit to a lifelong study of the canonical writings.

Arnaud Versluys, PhD, MD (China),
LAc Director, Institute of Classics in East Asian Medicine

Foreword

It is a great joy and honor for me to finally be writing this foreword to Z'ev Rosenberg's long-awaited first, but hopefully not last, book on Chinese medicine. So appropriately titled *Returning to the Source*, it is the encapsulation of a lifetime of studying and teaching and practicing Chinese medicine squarely in the tradition of the Chinese scholar-physicians that Z'ev aspires to follow. Spiced up liberally with enlightening quotations from Chinese medical literature of the past two thousand years, this book is a wake-up call for anybody interested in the past—*and* the future— of one of the longest and most effective paradigms of medicine in human history. Throughout the book, Z'ev makes convincing arguments in support of the need for a whole-hearted return to ancient wisdom to treat the ailments that plague our modern and post-modern bodies.

As many of the chapter titles suggest (e.g., "The Technician and the Scholar-Physician," "Ecological Medicine," "The Perfect Storm,"), this book is not afraid to address some thorny issues in our profession head on. Most importantly, this book is a warning against the ever-present danger of losing the true essence of the ancient wisdom by absorption into the dominant paradigm of modern biomedicine in the name of integration. As Z'ev points out throughout the book, this is already happening all too frequently in many institutional settings of Chinese medicine practice and education, both in China and the West. In contrast to the disconnection from life through modern technology that is found in modern biomedicine and our culture at large, Z'ev emphasizes such relevant aspects of Chinese medicine as vitalism, holism and resonance, balance, moderation, preventative medicine, and self-healing. This book convincingly argues that Chinese medicine, by "returning to the source," can provide elegant and innovative answers to our modern problems if we only allow it to stand on its own. His book offers a host of clinical examples to support this point.

For many reasons, my favorite chapter is perhaps the one titled "Ecological Medicine," which can be seen as a summary of the first few chapters of the "Plain Questions" (Su Wen) in the *Yellow Emperor's Inner Classic* (Huangdi Neijing). In this chapter, Z'ev expresses with perfect clarity a fundamental attitude that I could not agree with more: "For those of us who are committed to understanding and applying the medical teachings of the Han dynasty foundational texts, it is imperative that we study, teach, and live the principles found in these texts and let them guide our medical practices." Over the past dozen years or so, I have exchanged countless emails and phone calls and conversations with Z'ev, including a most delightful week-long herb walk in the mountains of New Mexico, exploring the connections between the ancient texts and our modern lives. Whether relaxing in the healing waters of Agua Caliente, poking around along the river banks off a random highway in pursuit of who knows what plant treasures, sipping tea in refined composure, jumping into action to alleviate a fellow human's suffering with sagely and compassionate advice, pouring over ancient dictionaries and materia medica literature, or discussing an obscure passage in the *Yellow Emperor's Inner Classic*, Z'ev loves this medicine with every nook and cranny of his heart, mind, and body. His writings are a perfect reflection of his teachings and practice thereof.

I have always been struck by Z'ev's boundless curiosity and enthusiasm for learning about other medicines and ways of healing in the largest sense of that word. This dedication has resulted in a deep and extensive erudition in many histories and traditions far beyond his specialty of Chinese medicine, and in a lifetime of practical experience as a dedicated clinical practitioner of classical Chinese medicine with an open mind to other healing modalities. This book is the fruit of a rich lifetime of learning, practicing, and teaching medicine, with a focus on traditional China. As such, it draws on Z'ev's extensive knowledge of medical history in China and his appreciation for the many contributing streams of knowledge in the transmission of Chinese medicine through the centuries. In addition, his views on medicine and healing are informed by his studies in other systems of medicine, from Greco-Arabic, Ayurvedic, and Tibetan medicine to contemporary biomedicine, as well as medical anthropology, philosophy, cosmology, and literature.

For those readers who have been fortunate to spend time in Z'ev's company, whether he happened to be your teacher, mentor, physician, friend, or colleague, you know that he means every word he has written in this book and has been applying the principles stated in these pages with utmost sincerity in both his personal and professional life. For those of you who do not know him personally, this book can provide a glimpse into his work and life. In the following pages, you will discover a powerful distillation of the key messages from the ancient Chinese medical classics, as relevant today as they were two thousand years ago, from harmonizing heaven and earth in a cosmological sense to a sustainable lifestyle of moderation and regulation, promoting self-healing by awakening the "internal pharmacy," and restoring a dynamic equilibrium in the process of qi transformation in accordance with the cycles of yin-yang and five phases. It is my sincere hope that this book will convince all readers of the need to let Chinese medicine thrive on its own terms, in the spirit of the ancient Han dynasty classics, instead of being swallowed up and subsumed by "integration" into the dominant biomedical paradigm. By "returning to the source," we may discover not only a fascinating history of the past but a way forward to solve the many problems that are currently threatening the co-existence of heaven, earth, and humanity.

Please read this book slowly and take its message seriously.

Sabine Wilms PhD
Whidbey Island, Washington,
August 27, 2017

Acknowledgements

Z'ev and Daniel wish to thank Micah Arsham, LAc, for her contributions to the foundations of this book early on. She spent many hours researching many years of Z'ev's journals for material, and edited early versions of the information in this book.

Introduction: Setting the Stage for Our Discussion

Classical Chinese medicine is based on a practical philosophy; it is a way of life and nurturing one's health, and also has many therapeutic modalities. There is no conflict between its practical application, and as a meditation on the natural world through natural science. This vision has sustained generations of great physicians, and produced many medical texts that were many years ahead of their time. Study in this system is concurrent with practice, they inspire and inform each other. The *rú yī* 儒醫/scholar-physician, is the pinnacle of a medicine that is a profession, a daily practice, a study regimen, an immersion in life, an expression of compassion, and so much more.

Having studied and practiced this medicine for most of my life, this book is inspired by my endless curiosity to study the sources of this vast medical tradition, a medicine that we've just begun to discover in the West. While modalities such as acupuncture are being embraced, we have not yet fully uncovered what the ancient sages of the Han dynasty had revealed as a crucial understanding and potential cure for the waves of poor health that increasingly engulf the world's population. This requires an investment from people in terms of cultivating their own health, beginning with education and a new ecological awareness of the bioregions in which we live. Chinese medicine is an approach that, above all, prevents illness, and when illness arises, the physician works in harmony with nature and the laws of the universe to dislodge the disease from the body, mind, and spirit. Our infatuation with the modern and the new has blinded us to the possibility that ancient societies, such as that in China during the Warring States period and Han dynasty, may have had a fully developed, ecologically inspired health science that has endured for over two thousand years. While we live in the 21st century, we should never forget that our future is bound up in our history, our roots, our soil, our cultures, and, of course, in the timelessness of spirituality that informs the renewal of life in our precious world.

The code, the essence of this perspective, can be found specifically in the classical texts of the *Su wen*, Chapters 1–6, and additionally in the *Ling shu, Nan jing, Shang han lun*, and the writings of prominent physicians from Zhong Zhongjing to Zhang Jingyue. These texts contain blueprints for attaining ideal health through meditating on the perceived patterns of heaven and earth, and then putting these principles into practice in daily life. With this compass, we can then see how even the most complicated diseases have developed out of original, simple causative factors.

After many years of study and reflection on Chinese medicine, I am convinced that the health of humanity is dependent on the health of the living Earth and of human society. In Chinese medicine, if one phase is out of balance, so other things are off their proper, physiological course. Thus, Wang Bing writes in his commentary of the *Su wen*, Chapter 3, "If the guard qi, the camp qi, and to the qi of the depots and palaces are out of balance, each of them may cause a disease."[1] Chinese medicine is nothing if not about relationships among various parts; it describes an ecological system, wherein parts are always related to the whole, and the wellness of the individual is bound to the well-being of society and nature. The *Nan jing* tells us that the physician heals the

1   Unschuld and Tessenow 2011: 65

diseases of society, and without this, many illnesses cannot be rectified. Medicine is also a way of life, and the classical Chinese medical texts such as the *Huang Di nei jing Su wen* teach us how to prevent illness by presenting principles of living in accordance with natural laws, and this is illustrated clearly in the first three chapters of the *Su wen*. These principles can be extended to agriculture, the environment, architecture and all human endeavors. Technology is simply the natural expression of human creativity and awareness, and when done harmoniously with natural law, it is a great aid to human life.

Z'ev Rosenberg
San Diego, September 2017

CHAPTER I

PHILOSOPHY AND MEDICAL EDUCATION
The Missing Piece

Man is a part of the world, and if we wish to understand his aim and activity, and use and place, then we must first know the purpose of the whole world, so that it will become clear to us what man's aim is, as well as the fact that man is necessarily a part of the world, in that his aim is necessary for realizing the ultimate purpose of the world.

Al Farabi[1]

Philosophy must not only be reinstated in Chinese medical studies, but must also be the very basis of any enlightened curriculum. Until a few decades ago, MD physicians and other service-related professionals received a broad liberal arts education, including philosophy. Today's students in Chinese medical schools need to be immersed in Asian philosophy and culture along with an Asian language (at the very least, medical Chinese or Japanese) in order to understand how the venerable medicine of Asia developed from the world view of these great civilizations. Specifically, yin/yang, five phase theory, and channel theory all developed from the specific cosmology of China that was the basis of the Jin and Han dynasties, and all that followed until the 20th century. This cosmology was

---

1   Mahdi 2001: 79

based on the *Yi jing* and Confucian classics, and was expressed in Chinese culture, politics, technology, and medicine.

It is also helpful to understand how Western philosophy, religion, and science developed throughout history. The work of Maimonides, the great Muslim philosophers (Al Farabi, Ibn Sina), and Aristotle nurtured the world view that predominated in classical Western sciences and philosophy.

Chinese medicine, like Ayurveda, Greco-Arabic medicine (*tibb-i-unani*), and Tibetan medicine, are "whole systems" medicines, including longevity and health cultivation, lifestyle, exercise regimens, physical manipulation, dietetics, and internal medicine. The West has quickly adapted acupuncture as a modality, largely because of its great successes in stress reduction, pain relief, and the familiarity of Westerners with surgical techniques (which it resembles, but in a much less invasive manner). However, in Chinese medical texts, internal or herbal medicine is 80 percent of the professional practice of medicine. This is not to denigrate acupuncture in any way— it is essential and especially important in the high-stress 21st century—but without its essential theory as outlined in the *Su wen* and *Ling shu*, it is reduced to a technique, watered down and reduced in its potential effectiveness.[2]

"Full strength" Chinese medicine can reveal to us in many cases the origins of human illness, and it can view the progression of disease states from possible origins. Chinese medicine as presented in the Han dynasty (and later) medical classics can potentially be a guiding light for the future development of world medicine; for example, see the new frontiers of genomics and systems biology and medicine as

---

2   By not understanding source principles outlined in such texts as the *Su wen*, *Ling shu*, *Jia yi jing* and *Nan jing*, the acupuncture practiced today suffers from the limitations of empiricism; in other words, using a specific point for a symptom, techniques for pain or musculoskeletal disorders. The full potential of acupuncture/moxibustion has not been realized in our present era, and the multiple models used to practice it from microsystems (ear, abdominal, hand) to biomedical/neurological approaches are far removed from their original understanding.

modern developments of what traditional cultures always practiced as systems sciences applied to medicine.[3]

We need textbooks in schools but we need to go beyond them and learn the operating system of Chinese medicine that is not taught in school. We are not really taught how yin and yang work or how the five phases work. Unless you are in a classically oriented school, you don't learn what defines defense qi, or construction qi, ministerial fire, or sovereign fire (in the heart). You don't learn about the theories of Li Dong-yuan or Zhu Dan-xi, which help us understand how autoimmune diseases develop. We need these theories to help us understand the complicated cases that we see in modern clinical practice. There is only one English language textbook on autoimmune disease and traditional Chinese medicine (TCM), and another on lupus and TCM, and both of them are very biomedically oriented. Because of this, both texts use very large formulas with cold, bitter, draining ingredients in them. American patients would find many of these formulas difficult to digest. Many of these formulas are toxic and potentially harmful. Modern, integrated TCM books such as these rely largely on a biomedical understanding of the body, or at best looking at autoimmune disease through a *wēn bìng* 溫病/warm disease lens. And if you don't have the principles I've mentioned, it is difficult to understand how to treat this rising tide of very complex disorders. Only by studying these theories can we understand why the body attacks itself, creating feedback loops of destructive symptoms.

To move away from the philosophical foundations of Chinese medicine, to water it down to be more "appealing" to Westerners is a great disservice to the public. And the first step in re-establishing its historical grandeur is to move away from an education based on data and technique rather than deep understanding of theory. As the physician thinks, so they practice. By immersing oneself in the Han dynasty world

---

3   See Institute of Systems Biology, www.systemsbiology.org

view of synchronicity, one begins to view one's patients as microcosmic expressions of the grand order of nature. From this perspective, illness is seen as an aberration of the laws of nature, and the role of the physician is to be as much a teacher, as much an applier of technique, in treating the body and mind in such a manner to restore dynamic equilibrium. The acupuncture and moxibustion techniques, herbal prescriptions and other clinical strategies are all expressions of sophisticated medical philosophy applied to the problems of the day, but are still applicable to modern conditions and diseases. Local conditions may change, but timeless principles do not.

CHAPTER II

ECOLOGICAL MEDICINE
The Heart of the *Su wen*
Medical Philosophy

The body ecologic

Recently, several scientists have viewed the human organism as part of a larger environmental body, one that is connected to other animals, plant life, seasons, climate, and recently the vast, invisible world of bacteria, viruses, molds, and fungi that interact with and inhabit us. This ecological point of view can be traced in the West to such early scientists as physiologist Claude Bernard, who coined the term *milieu interieur* and emphasized its importance in maintaining health. Greco-Arabic medicine's great physicians, such as Galen, Hippocrates, Ibn Sina, and Ibn Rushd, all taught the importance of balancing the humors and elements (earth, water, fire, air, blood, phlegm, yellow bile, and black bile). The revolution in medicine began with such figures as Louis Pasteur, who in the 19th century discovered the significance of specific pathogens, especially bacteria, in creating infectious disease. He pioneered the use of chemicals and minerals to attack them, as did Paul Erlich, with the use of mercury and other toxic chemicals. This trajectory culminated with the discovery of antibiotics in the 20th century. What originally appeared as a 'miracle drug' became problematic, as overuse of broad-spectrum antibiotics in animal feed for livestock and routine use in children and adults began to distort the ecological balance of microorganisms in the human biome. In the words of Gunapala Dharmasiri, in *The Nature of Medicine*:

> One of the greatest disasters that Western medicine has brought upon humanity is the creation of the science of antibiotics. It is true that at the beginning it worked and looked like a blessing. But the West did not have a correct philosophy of life and world to become aware of its deadly implications for the humans and the environment. Geoffrey Cannon, who has done extensive research into the field of antibiotics, writes: "In effect, antibiotics are pesticides used on people."[1]

Recently we have seen the development of superbugs, bacteria that actually eat antibiotics as they evolve according to laws of survival of the fittest. If a patient doesn't finish a course of antibiotics, there is a danger that hardy bacteria will complicate and lengthen the course of disease. Of course, if an antibiotic is given to a patient with a viral infection, it will definitely lengthen the course of disease and weaken the patient's defenses. The use of antibiotic handsoaps, and the feeding of antibiotics to animals only increases this problem.

Humanity is part of an ecological continuum, which in Han dynasty thought is the interface between heaven and earth. Human beings have had great power, through our technology, to influence our planet, but the side-effects of our technologies have led to the consumption of the yin aspect of earth (waterways have been dammed and polluted, forests and soil have been spoiled, while fossil fuels—which are like the essence (jīng 精) of the earth—have been exploited). The earth's ecosystems have shifted in new directions that until now were not apparent to the majority of people. China today would be unrecognizable by the Han dynasty philosopher-kings. We have gone from being stewards of the earth to destroyers of

---

1   Dharmasiri 1997: 47

the earth. Tragically, both Western capitalism and Chinese communism see the earth as a resource to be exploited. The struggle with nature is central to human survival. But in destroying the earth, we destroy our very foundation in the world.

However, once we breach the limits of sustainability, humanity starts to poison its air, water and soil, and as a direct result our food, water, air, and the natural medicines of the plant, animal, and mineral kingdoms are likewise tainted. Ironically, modern China has also led the way on the fast-track to 21st-century technological and industrialized culture, with its resulting malasdies and environmental destruction. Modern biomedicine, heavily dependent on advanced technology when compared with traditional medical systems, is a two-sided phenomenon that both can save lives and destroy health, sometimes simultaneously. Heroic drugs (that are often toxic) are widely overused. They diminish not only the innate natural healing power of an individual, his correct qi (*zhèng qì* 正氣), but they also degrade the environment. Overuse of antibiotics strip-mines the gastrointestinal system of its beneficial flora (bacteria that help digest our food and protect us from unhealthy bacteria and viruses). Genetically modified organisms, specifically foods, which are even more heavily sprayed with pesticides and fertilizer, destroy the delicate balance of plant and soil, and potentially alter the genetic code of our food supply to unknown ends. The same fertilizers and pesticides destroy the soil, while mono-culturing crops destroys diversity of plant life, obliterates forests and wild animals, and pollutes and depletes water supplies. One may also consider that medical advances (such as overuse of vaccines, antibiotics, fertility drugs, and such procedures like *in vitro* fertilization) potentially weaken future generations of humanity, for they bypass natural selection to an extreme degree.

Just as our environment changes, so too does the environment of our bodies. In his recent book, *An Epidemic of Absence* (2013), Moises Velasquez-Manoff explains that by losing contact with what he calls the ecosystem's "superorganism," i.e. the soil and its natural microorganisms, we imperil our immune systems, which leads to allergies and other autoimmune disorders. In the book, Velasquez-Manoff describes his personal battles with autoimmune alopecia and eczema, which led him to investigate the use of implantation with parasites for both himself, and in the treatment of patients with a wide range of autoimmune disorders from lupus to Crohn's disease. He reports in his book of successful cases in remission for various lengths of time, some of them dramatic. But what is most important in his research is revealing how the industrial and technological revolutions have transformed human ecology on a massive scale. The majority of humanity have left their farmer and hunter roots to become city dwellers. Nowhere has this trend seen a more dramatic acceleration than in China, where hundreds of millions of peasants have been moved (or have chosen to move) from the land to large cities, many built from scratch. This has occurred alongside a vast increase of toxic chemicals released into the environment, and this problem is compounded by the indiscriminate ingestion of antibiotics, steroids, and other pharmaceuticals by both humans and domesticated animal species. Over the centuries, large-scale environmental disruptions have occurred. Wars, famines, droughts, floods, and extreme weather have led to epidemics and disruptions in the immune system. However, human beings were able to adapt over time because they lived relatively close to nature, so the vast microflora both inside and outside us adjusted and adapted to these changes.

The root of the problem is the same for the individual as for society in general. Among the most significant issues of our time in public health is the subtle, often hidden destruction of the microbiome. Just as the complexity and diversity of nature has been compromised by clear-cutting forests, the loss of countless animal and plant species, urbanization, and factory farming (with miles of single crops replacing complex prairie bioregions), so we have cheated the varied, and unseen, microbiome of our own bodies. The sterilization of hospitals, homes, and public places by antibiotic handsoaps, denatured foods, crop spraying, and countless other technological alterations have led to changes in the universal microbiome. As we find new innovative ways to forestall death through surgeries, miracle drugs, vaccines, and replacement body parts, we also replace former killers in the developed world such as tuberculosis, sepsis, and smallpox with epidemics of autoimmune diseases, allergies, eczema, and gluten intolerance, while other subtle and hard-to-understand illnesses remain outside our ability to bring them under control. There is clear evidence that our modern post-industrial lifestyles have impoverished our environment, and that we are now living in a greatly altered world of our own creation (one that has generated new environmental crises that we could not have imagined even a few decades ago). Additionally, it has created new health crises due to the concurrent relationship of the internal environment to the external one.

Ecological medicine must be based on the grounding of humanity in its relation with heaven (including cosmic formative forces, astronomy, the location and rotation of sun, moon, planets, stars, solar winds, and gravitational fields) and earth (including ecosystems, seasons, climate, flora, fauna, winds, humidity, pressure changes, body type, food, and social ecology). It seeks to harmonize humans with the natural environment in order to maximize health and prevent disease. This perspective recognizes that humankind has been greatly altered by modern medicine, specifically, such developments as the incubation of "preemies," vaccines, the overuse of anti-biotics (including sterilization and pasteurization), our lack of exposure to soil and micro-organisms, and, significantly, *in vitro* fertilization, which allows older adults and infertile people to have children. The genie is out of the bottle, and we have changed the genome of not only human beings, but of our own food supply through genetic engineering. Other than an environmental holocaust, it doesn't seem likely that all of this can or will be reversed.

The seminal *Su wen* chapters: a blueprint for human and ecological health

The essential first three chapters of the *Huang Di nei jing Su wen* set the stage for the core principles of Chinese medicine. These opening chapters contain the compass of life and medicine; the text reveals the equations that allow us to see how far we've deviated from the principles of life. As Wang Bing explains in his commentary of chapter 3 in the *Su wen*:

> If one's desires cannot fatigue one's eyes, if the evil of lewdness cannot confuse one's heart, if no recklessness causes fatigue, this is "clarity and purity." Because of one's clarity and purity, the flesh and interstice [structures] are closed and the skin is sealed tightly. The true and proper qi guards the interior and no depletion evil intrudes... Those that are "clear and pure" follow the order/sequence of the four seasons, ...they do not cause fatigue through reckless behavior, and rising and resting follow certain rules. As a result, their generative qi is never exhausted and they are able to preserve their strength forever.[2]

Many modern practitioners of Chinese medicine criticize the seminal first three chapters of the *Su wen* as "fantasy" about a world that no longer exists, of sages living in perfect harmony with the way (*dào* 道). The *Su wen* describes it as an ideal, as a way of living that even at the time of the *Huang Di nei jing* was long past. In chapter 1 of the *Su wen* Huang Di asks Qi Bo:

> The people of high antiquity, in [the sequence of] spring and autumn, all exceeded one hundred years. But in their movements and activities there was no weakening. As for the people of today, after one half of a hundred years, the

---

2   Unschuld and Tessenow 2011: 72

movements and activities of all of them weaken. Is this because the times are different? Or that the people have lost this [ability]?

Qi Bo responded:

The people of high antiquity, those who knew the Way, they modeled [their behavior] on yin and yang.... [Their] eating and drinking was moderate. [Their] risings and resting had regularity. They did not tax [themselves] with meaningless work. Hence, they were able to keep physical appearance and spirit together, and to exhaust the years [allotted by] heaven. Their life span exceeded one hundred years before they departed.[3]

What many people don't comprehend from the passage is that the *Su wen* presents the principles for the practice of ecological medicine, based on living in harmony with natural law and its influences on the intricacies of human health. This has been known since ancient times, first mentioned in the Mawangdui manuscripts, as nourishing life (*yǎng shēng* 養生). The ideal way of life attributed to the sages is based on the intrinsic harmony of heaven (sky) and earth, and the human being as an intermediary between these poles of existence. So right at the beginning of Chinese history, we are seeing that the human being has a profound influence on the world around them.

In modern times, the predominating dogma(s) in modern science, on the one hand, are that nature is unconscious, working according to Darwinian mechanisms that push survival and adaption forward. On the other hand, there are the religious fundamentalists who believe that such phenomena as climate change are a hoax, and free-market evangelists who believe that energy companies should be deregulated and allowed to despoil the environment in the name of economic need and job growth. Nowhere is this problem more acute than in mainland China, as we discussed above. The closest modern

3   Unschuld and Tessenow 2011: 30–33

theory to that discussed in the ancient texts that I could find from a scientist is James Lovelock and Lynn Margulis' Gaia Theory,[4] which states that the earth is a living being that responds to our activities. One of the great sea changes of the scientific revolution in the West was the complete repudiation of what is called the vitalist principle (the concept of a life force in creation that animates all living and sentient beings), replaced by a more mechanistic view of life. In my opinion, this is the biggest rift between Western and Chinese medicine. And to the degree that Chinese medicine abandons so-called vitalism, it moves far from its Han dynasty sources.

Algorithms of disconnection: deviation from the *Nan jing* 難經 and *Su wen* 素問 matrix of health

Within the amazing technological advances of modern biomedicine, from which we all benefit and literally live with, combined with the advances in modern agriculture and animal husbandry, an equal and opposite devolution has occurred in the nature of mankind itself. Because we have lived inside this revolution for a few generations now, few of us have been able to step outside and see another perspective to the status of human beings on this planet. In the last hundred years or so, we have passed a point where we are almost entirely subject to nature and its patterns, and have entered an era where exploding population growth, expectations of affluence, and technology are altering nature itself. Yet we are often unable to see how drastically the earth has changed. Today we cross time zones, traveling through the world in hours by jet plane when it used to take weeks of long, perilous journeys by foot, horse, camel, or ship. In doing so we have altered our circadian rhythms. When we work under artificial light on computer screens, we alter the amount of stimulus to our eyes and brains, and impact our normal sleep cycles. When we eat refined,

---

4   For more information on Gaia Theory refer to www.gaiatheory.org/overview

devitalized, and now genetically modified food, we alter our metabolism and microbiome, and when we put ever-stronger chemical pesticides on our produce, we poison ourselves. The climate is changing dramatically, human waste is building up in oceans, rivers, and in the soil, and water supplies are drying up.

The *Yellow Emperor's Internal Classic: Simple Questions* (*Huang Di nei jing Su wen*) as we've previously discussed, embodies an ecological vision that is the cornerstone of medicine, specifically in *Su wen* Chapters 1–5. *Spiritual Pivot* (*Ling shu* 64) discusses constitutional types based on climatic origins, size, shape, length of limbs and torso, qualities of personality, vitality, intellect and physical strength, and regional variations based on utilization of caloric heat circulated by the ministerial fire (*xiàng huǒ* 相火), "inhabiting the life gate, liver, gallbladder and triple burner (*sān jiāo* 三焦)." This constitutional legacy of human beings, who were forced for millennia to adapt to environmental and weather and climatic conditions, has been greatly altered since the industrial revolution, largely unseen to us all. Now we control our climate through air conditioning and central heating, we ship foods that are out of season across the world rather than has access only to seasonal or locally grown produce. The relative ease and comfort of modern life have changed us. No longer is "exercise" dictated by the sheer need for survival (such as farming, chopping wood, building homes, or travel), but by the need for activity, building muscle, or modifying one's appearance. Often this is a reaction to the extreme sedentary nature of modern life. Appetite for food is often dictated not by survival, but advertising, addiction to extreme flavors, or by emotional needs.

Using the *Su wen* as the foundation for my understanding of a new ecological medicine in the 21st century, I've classified all of these factors as "algorithms of disconnection." By returning to the Han dynasty renaissance of medicine (which modern Chinese people need just as much as the West), and understanding the principles of yin and yang, seasonal transformations, influence of climate, and nourishing life (*yǎng shēng* 養生), we can understand the degree of disconnection we have from a normal and healthy life. We can take steps to rectify this damage through lifestyle, regulation of work, exercise and rest, improving diet, harmonizing emotions, and seeking Chinese medical treatment to harmonize the various humors and generating forces in our bodies and minds.

Two thousand years later, the words that are at the very beginning of the *Su wen* resonate with our present health crisis in post-industrial culture. But how can we apply these ancient principles of moderation and regulation to our modern dilemma? We can do this by deep study of the classical texts such as the *Su wen* and, specifically, the *Nan jing*, which lays the groundwork in its 81 difficulties (chapters) for understanding the baseline of health and deviation from the principles and factors that influence the ebb and flow of health, namely: season, time of day, constitution and body type, climate, patterns of work and rest, taxation, emotional equilibrium. These are the influences that allow the channels and viscera-bowel systems to work together harmoniously. Our modern, post-industrial civilization deviates from natural law in several significant ways, and these differences certainly affect our overall health. These patterns of deviation from the ancient norm and ideal include particularly modern phenomena that are the result of a fast-paced, globalized world: taxation, dietary factors, environmental damage, disease suppression, emotional overload, overstimulation of the senses, counterintuitive work schedules, and living out of sync with one's constitution.

Regarding taxation, an alarming percentage of Americans have chronic sleep deprivation. Overworking with inadequate sleep can damage internal body clocks, opening the door to chronic, autoimmune disease. Dietary factors exacerbate this problem. It is evident that as industrialized junk food spreads through developing countries, the rates of obesity, diabetes, and cancer increase exponentially. The further we deviate from eating foods in season that are locally grown and organic and ideally prepared with minimal processing, the more chronic disease increases. Damage to the environment has been discussed: the air, water, soil, and food are laced with chemicals from fertilizers and pesticides that are potentially carcinogenic. Remembering that even 60 years ago most food was organic and unprocessed, this recent experiment with industrializing the food supply, compounded now with over-hybridization and genetic modifications, is so ubiquitous that few see the damage it has done.

Similar to the alterations caused by changes to our food supply, the suppression of disease by modern medicine has changed the ways in which our bodies function. We have powerful interventions: pharmaceutical drugs, surgeries, and radiation treatments that can save lives when used appropriately. But these same treatments, when used at the wrong time or for more benign conditions, cause great damage to mind and body. A prime example is the overuse of antibiotics for routine respiratory infections, a vast majority of which are viral and do not respond to these drugs. Physicians and patients alike demand these treatments, and have become used to their side-effects and suppressive nature, that often relieve the branch (biāo 標) symptoms, but fail to treat the root (běn 本) factors. Often, this approach drives disease to a deeper level in the body, usually the yin viscera. Deeply set diseases (such as those of the yin layers of the body) often do not cause acute symptoms, but the patient slowly manifests disease from within. For example, anti-hypertensive drugs will indeed lower blood pressure, but without lifestyle and diet changes and stress management, the blood pressure will rise back to its original level even after taking these drugs for several years.

Another pathogenic factor that is exacerbated by modern life is emotional overload and overstimulation of our senses. In contrast to how many of us live today, people in pre-war Europe lived in the same village all their lives and knew all their neighbors, people with whom they were forced to cooperate in order to survive and fulfill their needs. They lived in the same home, married and rarely divorced, had their extended families living nearby, and saw the same sun rise and set over the same landscape for an entire lifetime. In contrast, today, people move all over the world, travel through multiple time zones, and are often not close with their families (which are often fragmented by divorce). The average Westerner has had multiple intimate relationships and breakups, and this increase of heartbreak and emotional upheaval has an impact on health.

The geographic upheaval of our lives also reflects on our constitution, as constitutional types are now jumbled as we move from one region to another. Until perhaps a hundred years ago, few people travelled extensively. While historically there have always been large population shifts, due to drought, famine, or war, people generally lived close to their birth place, ate locally grown and raised foodstuffs, and developed in synchronicity with the local environment. *Ling shu* 64 discusses constitutional types in depth, showing how people's bodies evolved to deal with specific environmental conditions. Northern people were shorter, with broader waists, thicker skin and more body fat; they responded to environmental cold by producing internal heat from high caloric foods and a thick skin and fat layer to keep the heat inside. In *Su wen* 3, it says that one should not sweat one's vitality away in winter, as one loses vital heat and weakens one's kidneys. In southern regions, people are slimmer, generally taller, with less body fat and a thinner skin layer with pores that open easily to release sweat, from the yang heat of the stronger southern sun, which coaxes excessive heat from a person's core out to the exterior.

Counterintuitive work schedules are rampant in America, as well as other countries that keep up with a global economy. Having observed medical schools and their schedules, let's just say that people are forced to ignore their circadian rhythms in terms of sleep, waking, eating, elimination, naps, exercise, and other essentials to maintain health. Students of all types are forced to compete in memorizing data by cramming, staying up all night with the help of stimulant drugs, then using tranquilizers to sleep. This lifestyle slowly and certainly damages one's health. It is no surprise that many college students fall apart physiologically and emotionally on campus, when no limits to sleep, partying, alcohol, and drugs are imposed, along with a crushing schedule of classes and study. In contrast, the ancient medical texts recommend a regular living schedule that harmonizes with seasonal and daily rhythms to maintain health and safeguard against disease.

Using the pulse, abdominal and channel palpation, questioning, complexion (sè 色), and our other diagnostic tools, we can calculate how far a person has deviated from the golden mean described in these classical texts, and for how long. The *Nan jing* specifically uses a mathematical model that can be deciphered through repetitive study, in terms of yin-yang, five phase theory, and the eight extraordinary vessels. The *Shang han lun* presents a six-channel progression of exterior environmental evils from the surface to the interior of the body, one that draws from the *Nei jing*. Even though today we have traveled far from this golden mean, we can reintroduce lifestyle strategies and treatments to reactivate internal body clocks, and harmonize with our environment to restore ground rules for health.

Life ends and begins again: musings on cycles of life and the *Su wen*

We can read the *Su wen* largely as an ecological manual that provides the foundational principles on which a healthy society can function. It teaches us how to live with the seasons, about constitutional types, about variances in diet, climate and living conditions and how they influence human health and disease. The Han dynasty medical classics, including the *Nan jing, Shen nong ben cao jing*, and *Shang han za bing lun*, give us a broad palate of principles based on mathematical models of inquiry into nature and time. These texts teach us how to understand nature's transformations through specific embedded cycles of years, seasons, months, and days. They teach us to live harmoniously in this world in the most ecological way possible. Ancient Chinese scholars accessed this world as their laboratory. They expressed their findings in the very structure of the Chinese language, which was originally a pictographic language that conveyed visual and cognitive information in the characters. Medicine (*yī xué* 醫學) developed out of this model that views life as an unbroken chain of interconnected plant, mineral, animal, and human communities. As in every other human discipline, from the arts (calligraphy), architecture, agriculture, and metallurgy, to the very structure of family and society, the principles of yin and yang encoded in the *Classic of Change* (*Yi jing*) were the root of the understanding and application of a practical cosmology.

Modern China has strayed from its roots and traded the *Yi jing* for "Mr. Science." It demands that its native medicine be based on modern science, and we can only expect that what is called Chinese medicine today may easily slip away and be absorbed into biomedicine. For those of us who are committed to understanding and applying the medical teachings of the Han dynasty foundational medical texts, it is imperative that we study, teach and live the principles found in these texts and let them guide our medical practices. What modern physicians, both Eastern and Western, find difficult to understand is how medical texts written two thousand years ago can possibly guide clinical practice in the 21st century, a time when modern medicine is changing by the week due to new discoveries in research.

What isn't immediately apparent is that modern bio-medicine has not changed its principles since the late 19th century. It is still based largely on anatomy and physiology, pharmaceutics, and molecular biology. While there are discoveries such as new drugs (although drug discovery seems to be slowing down) and changes in treatment protocols, little has changed outside the technological veneer. Chinese medicine, as we discussed earlier, is based on ecological principles, such as visceral manifestation (*zàng xiàng* 臟象) theory, which states that internal functions of the internal structures and viscera can be viewed in changes on the surface of the body. It would be a betrayal of the generations of physicians who kept these teachings alive through a vast, thriving medical literature, including case histories, to allow this medical tradition to be slowly absorbed into biomedicine in the name of integration.

True integration means mutual respect and interaction between two fully developed medical systems. They will be able to cross-fertilize even more in the future as biomedicine incorporates new "systems biology" and "systems medicine" models, which are less reductionist and more open-ended; these models embrace transformation and change in a way not unlike the textual foundation of Chinese medicine. This is a much better option than what Paul Unschuld has called the "Tibetanization of Chinese medicine."[5] He uses the example of monasteries in Tibet that serve as tourist attractions and have exotic edifices, but whose practices are slowly dying as the number of practicing meditators decreases (due to lack of exposure to the younger generations of Tibetans who are discouraged from its practice). It is the same with Chinese medicine in China, where the empirical data about formulas and diseases remains, but acupuncture and moxibustion have largely been reduced to a form of physical therapy. Pulse and traditional diagnostic systems have been de-emphasized in favor of modern technological screening, and the younger generation are no longer educated in systematic correspondence or in a world view that is noticeably different from that of modern science imported from the West.

---

5   Lecture presented by Paul Unschuld at Pacific Symposium 2003 in California, San Diego

Here in the West, we are a very young profession, and what we have received in translation has already been integrated and watered down from China. Without the effort to understand Chinese medicine from its core, specific acupuncture techniques and point protocols will perhaps survive, but the use of herbal medicine, moxibustion, dietetics, and the unique diagnostics and perspective of Chinese medicine will disappear; few will notice its passing. This would be a great tragedy.

CHAPTER III

CHINESE MEDICINE AND THE INTERNAL PHARMACY
The Body/Mind's Self-Healing Tools and Substances

When talking to both patients and other health care professionals, practitioners of Chinese medicine are often at a loss to describe how acupuncture and herbal medicine work, and how to distinguish them both from biomedicine and from other alternative therapies. In order to be able to contribute to the dialogue of modern-day health care, we need to understand these underlying principles and philosophy of Chinese medicine, as understood in its source texts. The foundations of Chinese medicine are to be found primarily in the Han dynasty medical classics such as the *Yellow Emperor's Classic of Internal Medicine* (*Huang Di nei jing Su wen* 黃帝內經), *Classic of Difficulties* (*Nan jing* 難經), and *Treatise on Cold Damage and Complex Diseases* (*Shang han za bing lun* 傷寒雜). They are expressed through the rubrics of systematic correspondence, such as yin-yang, five phases, defense and construction qi (*wèi qì* 衛氣 and *yíng qì* 營氣), channels and network vessels (*jīng luò* 經絡), and the complex terminology of the subject matter. Superficially immersing ourselves in the language of Western medicine will not aid us in understanding Chinese medicine; rather, through serious study, collaboration, and research, we can approach Chinese medicine on its own terms. We should also remember that until the early 20th century, all global medical systems such as Ayurveda, Greco-Arabic, and Tibetan medicine were based on mind-body systems and an emphasis on humors that still survives in the modern era. Even modern biomedicine retains influences from its roots in Greco-Arabic medicine, with its four elements and four humors (black bile, yellow bile, blood and phlegm).

Many years ago, I observed a panel discussion held by pharmacists at the University of California San Diego, who concluded that the future of medicine lies in what they called "the internal pharmacy." In other words, the next frontier in medicine will comprise techniques that use endogenous medicinal substances, rather than adding medicines from the outside. In this light, modern researchers have examined biofeedback, meditation, yoga, qi gong, natural remedies, and diet as methods of activating these powerful substances. The "internal pharmacy" is similar to what the 19th-century physiologist Claude Bernard called the *milieu interieur*, i.e. the internal environment or "terrain." Bernard explains that the internal environment is of paramount importance for one's health, as "the constancy of the internal environment (*milieu interieur*) is the essential condition for a free life."[1] This concept is still used today by French physicians. The "internal pharmacy" has incredibly sophisticated self-regulating mechanisms. The brain (along with the vital organs, endocrine glands, and nervous system) produces myriad substances which are the same or similar to many pharmaceutical drugs. Various opioid-like substances, steroids, painkillers, and hormones circulate continuously through the body, maintained in a very delicate balance by what we can call the "body/mind intelligence," a regulatory system that is still not well understood by any modern explanation. According to Neil Shubin, author of *The Universe Within*:

---

1   Bernard, Greene, Henderson and Cohen 2013: 24

We carry more than two trillion clocks inside of us. Our cellular clocks reside in the molecular machinery of DNA, which makes proteins that interact with one another and with DNA itself. Some combinations of these biological factors form a kind of molecular pendulum that swings back and forth between high and low levels of protein and gene activity, tuned to a virtual 24-hour day.[2]

In the 19th century, there was a debate between Louis Pasteur and Pierre Jacques Antoine Béchamp about the nature of disease. Louis Pasteur, of course, was famous for the discovery of infectious agents including bacteria, which he considered to be the prime cause of disease, while Pierre Jacques Antoine Béchamp considered imbalances of the *milieu interieur* to be the prime cause. Interestingly, on his death bed, Pasteur supposedly said that Béchamp was correct, but Pasteur's students went on to evangelize the doctrine of infectious disease agents with no regard for the patient's terrain or internal environment. It is "historical accidents" such as these that often lead to predominant trends in science. Of course, Pierre Jacques Antoine Béchamp was in full agreement with Claude Bernard's *milieu interieur.*

In Chinese medicine we understand these substances through their functional aspects as various expressions of qi, including *wèi qì* 衛氣/defense qi, *yíng qì* 營氣/construction qi, *jīng qì* 精氣/essential qi, *yuán qì* 原氣/source qi, and *zàng qì* 臟氣/visceral qi. These different qualities of qi, circulating and communicating in a grid of channels and network vessels, provide a framework to understand how the body and mind regulate themselves and maintain their equilibrium. Chinese medicine, in contrast to modern biomedicine, is based on binary principles established in such canonical texts as the *Classic of Change* (*Yi jing* 難經), and a holistic view of the universe in which human beings are an integral part. Human health is considered to be a reflection of an orderly universe,

---

2   Shubin 2013

and internal order reflects living with and adjusting to the external order of the universe. This is expressed through laws of season, climate, and environment, and adapting through clothing, diet, lifestyle, residence, moderated emotions, work, rest, and other human activities. The Chinese medical classics, such as the Han dynasty source text *Classic of Difficulties* (*Nan jing* 難經), with its 81 "difficulties", are clearly based on this principle. The purpose of diagnosis by pulse and palpation, theoretical application of yin-yang and five phase theory, and the application of needles and moxibustion treatment to channels and acupuncture holes aims to restore equilibrium to the dynamic systems represented by viscera and bowels, and channels and network vessels. What the *Nan jing* describes is a dynamic approach to a complex system, one in which the activation of self-healing mechanisms restores homeostasis.

The two main and most visible technologies of Chinese medicine are acumoxa therapy and internal (herbal) medicine. This is not to undervalue counseling, dietetics, therapeutic exercise, and lifestyle as essential components of Chinese medicine. But these therapeutic modalities are the most "active" and professional of Chinese medical interventions, and ones that can be readily studied as therapeutic interventions in their own right. Acupuncture and moxibustion as described in the *Yellow Emperor's Internal Classic: Simple Questions* (*Huang Di nei jing Su wen*), *Classic of Difficulties* (*Nan jing*), and *Divine Pivot* (*Ling shu*) are treatment modalities designed to restore equilibrium of channel flow between left and right, up and down, inside and outside. Most importantly, these adjustments recalibrate the body clocks that regulate so many functions (including digestion, sleep, activity, thought, hormonal secretions, emotional states, and blood circulation) and their timing. For example, one method of treating irregular menstrual periods is to utilize points along or coupled with the eight extraordinary vessels (*qí jīng bā mài* 奇經八脈), specifically the generating and controlling vessels (*chōng mài* 衝脈 and *rèn mài* 任脈). Thus, classical methods of acupuncture do not primarily focus on relieving symptoms, but rather they restore dynamic equilibrium to the body and mind by allowing self-healing mechanisms to take hold.

A terrain as it pertains to medicine is the landscape or environment in which specific patterns and phenomena occur. The view presented by Zhang Zhongjing in the *Treatise on Cold Damage (Shang han lun* 傷寒論*)*, and later developed by the authors of the warm disease current (*wēn bìng xué pài* 溫病學派), is a topographical one: they are both "immunological maps," or maps of responses to invasion by evil qi. The six-channel pattern differentiation (*liù jīng biàn zhèng* 六經辨證) describes a gradation of depth in the body, as it can be visualized as if laying out three-dimensional topographical maps of terrain illustrated by symptom patterns. In other words, *tài yáng* 太陽 or *shào yáng* 少陽 disease is a dynamic system in disequilibrium, and we introduce herbal treatment and acupuncture treatment to restore equilibrium. Even without attacks of evil qi, there are terrains of *tài yáng* 太陽, *yáng míng* 陽明, *shào yáng* 少陽 and so on associated with the amount of blood and qi in the channels, the parts of the body they influence, and emotional aspects that they control. Channels are multi-dimensional in this sense; they are not lines superimposed on the physical body. When the specific terrain of *tài yáng* 太陽, for example, becomes imbalanced and therefore ill (as in damage by wind), one rebalances the terrain with a herbal prescription or combination of acupuncture points to make the terrain inhospitable to *xié qì* 邪氣/evil qi (wind, in this case). The terrain strategy views disease as a moving target, and deals with not only the expulsion of evils (pathogens), but also with the idea of a dynamic balance and equilibrium among the various layers and components of the body, including emotional aspects.

By aiding transformation, the body takes care of itself, by resonantly aligning with heaven and earth what the body produces what it needs: *shào yīn* 少陰, *tài yáng* 太陽, and so on are movements of yin and yang between heaven and earth. The medicines in the *Treatise on Cold Damage and Miscellaneous*

Diseases (Shang han za bing lun 傷寒雜病論) are designed based on direction and movement: in many ways, the formulas are about qi transformation *(qì huà* 氣化*)* and not about material substances (tissues, blood, viscera, essence). Zhang Zhongjing's formulas are not vitamin supplements—they are agents of transformation. Hence Qi Bo explains the *Su wen,* Chapter 29:

> The spleen is earth and manages the center. It constantly promotes the growth of the other four viscera throughout the four seasons. With 18 days given for the spleen to manage, it is not allowed to rule one season. The spleen carries constantly the essence of stomach earth. Earth engenders the 10,000 things in accordance with heaven and earth. Hence the spleen reaches up to the head and down to the feet with no season for it to rule.[3]

Thus, the terrain of the body has first and foremost to do with earth. In Chinese medicine, this is the healthy functioning of the spleen and stomach. Many of the formulas listed in the *Shang han lun* include *tài yīn* 太阴/spleen supplementing medicinals (such as *dà zǎo* 大棗/jujube, *shēng jiāng* 生薑/fresh ginger, and *zhì gān cǎo* 炙甘草/honey fried licorice). The ability to digest the herbs is paramount. Through qi transformation, the body demonstrates its innate ability to produce what it needs. Herbal formulas, like acupuncture, are a natural overlay that directs earthly matter toward healthier patterns.

For the most part, Chinese medicine works with the existing tools of the patient's blood, qi, viscera, and channel system to resist and expel pathogens. Although there are toxic medicinal substances and powerful acumoxa treatments that do take a more militant approach to disease, it is more the exception than the rule. Although there was a school, the attack-evil current of thought *(gōng xié pài* 攻邪派*)* founded by Zhang Zi-he that focused on forcefully eliminating evils from the body, Zhang's approach never became mainstream. Systemic diseases, such

---

3   Li and Flaws 2004: 66

as cancer, are best treated by prevention, rather than by chemotherapy, radiation, and surgery, which take such a toll on patients, often killing them faster than the cancer does. W. Daniel Hillis, the famous physicist, was recently funded to start an institute to research systems approaches to cancer treatment at the University of Southern California.

> It's true that the human body is an amazing structure, but what's much more interesting is the process that builds it, that maintains it, modifies it. That's not really in the genes, it's in the conversation that's happening between all the parts of the body, and the conversation is happening within the little molecular machines within the cell, or between the cells in the body.
>
> But a systems disease like cancer, or an auto-immune disease, is a break down in the system, much more like a program bug. We would never think of debugging a computer by putting it into one of twelve categories, and doing something based on the category. Actually we do, it is kind of "help-desk debugging" that doesn't work very well in complex situations.[4]

So, what is equilibrium then, and how do patients attain it? In essence, the body remembers equilibrium that has been lost by habitual bias, i.e. by adapting to an unhealthy state. In other words, we get "stuck" in a habitual pattern that is less than ideal, and begin to self-medicate blindly with aspirin, alcohol, too much exercise, overeating, and other destructive behaviors. The strength of Chinese medicine is that it works not only on the physical body, or "architectural body," but also on what medical anthropologist Elisabeth Hsu calls the ecological and sentimental bodies. According to Hsu, the Han dynasty Chinese conceptualized the human body in terms of health and disease in a threefold manner: first, the architectural body: which is based on direction, depth, time and synchronization as expressed in the channel system; second, the ecological

---

4   Hillis 2010

body of tissues, fluids, and blood, ideally seen as "solid, firm, and polished like a fresh plant, with shiny glossy leaves and stems full of water." This solid body was seen to be an ideal receptacle of qi and its transformations; and third, perhaps most significantly, the sentimental body. The Han Chinese saw the five viscera (wŭ zàng 五臟) as receptacles of emotions and qi. Paraphrasing the Su wen, grief, fear, rage and anger harm the qi. As such, emotions in Chinese medicine are completely integrated with health and disease; when too extreme, they are considered part of pathology, and when balanced, are deemed an essential component of the healing process.

Our duty to patients is not to treat symptoms with simple "protocols," but rather to see clearly what made them ill in the first place and try to help them heal from within, if possible. Thus, as Elisabeth Hsu makes clear in her study of Chunyu Yi's memoir of 25 case histories, it is clearly laid out in the classic texts that we must enquire about emotions since the viscera are depositories of emotions and qi. Chunyu Yi's text is from the Han dynasty and accordingly focuses on the synchronicity between phenomena occurring inside the body—emotions— and the macrocosm of the greater environment. Dr. Chunyu diagnoses by palpating the vessels, and in his medical universe, the viscera are not primarily physiological entities but depots containing emotions and qi. He focuses on visceral qi and its specific qualities (color, scent, season, pulse image), and the primary disease factors are imbalanced emotions. As it says in Chapter 77 (Discourse on Expounding the Five Faults) of the Su wen:

> Whenever one wishes to diagnose a disease, it is essential to inquire about... whether he has experienced violent joy or suffering, or an initial joy followed by suffering. All this harms the essence qi. When the essence qi is exhausted and [its flow] interrupted, the physical body will be destroyed.[5]

---

5   Unschuld and Tessenow 2011: 668–669

Accordingly, Huang Di adds, "Separation and interruption, dense compactness and knotting, anxiety, fear, joy, and anger, [whether they let] the five depots (viscera) be empty and depleted and [whether they let] blood and qi lose their guardian [function], if the practitioner fails to know this, what art (of medicine) is there to speak of?"[6] It is quite an experience to look beyond the veil of Aristotelian causation (the finding of past factors that contribute to present illness) into an entirely synchronous world view without past or future, but only an eternal present. Studying Han dynasty texts opens one up to a world view that we've largely forgotten, but one that is essential to understand the foundation of Chinese medicine, for once without the overlay of our modern conceptions of reality.

Responsibility to the terrain of one's body has another meaning in Chinese culture, in the imperative to nourish one's life. In Confucian ethics, our body is a gift from our parents, and it is under our care and trust as long as we are alive. In addition, preserving our health is our obligation so that we may produce healthy offspring, who in turn will produce healthy offspring. In other words, health, like the environment, is in our trust for future generations. When we speak of genetics in the Chinese medical context, we need to go beyond the random yet fixed view that most modern people seem to have. Genetics is not a roll of random dice, but a process that can be influenced by many things, including diet, environment, emotions, our mating partners, and lifestyles. A new scientific discipline is epigenetics that investigates whether the genetic code is not a fixed, arbitrary grouping of genes, but rather that our programming can be influenced by all of these factors. Chinese medicine does not endorse rigid genetics unaffected by the environment or a person's lifestyle, that a human being was just a cipher of a blind mechanism. Another ancient medicine, Ayurveda, has similar ideas, namely, that parents have a responsibility to future generations, and if they

---

6   Unschuld and Tessenow 2011: 672–673

have any chronic illness, to do *panchakarma* therapy (with cleansing diet, herbs, steam baths, massage with oils, etc.) to clear their cells of the pathological factors. What our parents and previous generations thought, ate, the medicines they took, the events of their life, all were recorded into essence (*jīng* 精), sperm and ovum. But they are mutable, changeable, and part of a continuing stream that is never fixed or rigid in time and space.

In Chinese internal medicine, we primarily use poly-pharmacy (prescriptions that have multiple ingredients that work in concert). These herbal prescriptions can be said to treat not only presenting symptom patterns but the underlying terrain as well. Herbal prescriptions can be envisioned as complex external systems designed to interact with the internal environment in such a way that dynamic equilibrium is restored. Each ingredient of a prescription is chosen according to how it interacts with other ingredients to create a complex system that matches the specific pattern revealed through pattern differentiation (*biàn zhèng* 辯證). This approach also ensures that such relatively toxic medicinal substances such as *zhì fù zǐ* 制附子/prepared aconite root are always combined with medicinal substances such as *shēng jiāng* 生薑/fresh ginger root or *gān cǎo* 甘草/licorice root to reduce toxicity, in addition to the intensive processing (*páo zhì* 炮製) that medicinal grade aconite always undergoes before being used internally.

In the first definitive Chinese herbal text, *Shen nong ben cao jing* 神農本草經 (*The Divine Farmer's Materia Medica*), medicinal substances are divided into three grades: superior, middle, and inferior. Superior medicinal substances were those that had no side-effects and, like foods, could be consumed over an extended period with no harm. This included substances such as *dà zǎo* 大棗/jujube, *zhì gān cǎo* 炙甘草/honey prepared licorice root, and *rén shēn* 人參/Chinese ginseng, designed for nourishing life (*yǎng shēng* 養生). Middle-grade medicinal substances, which had mild side-effects and treated the personality and supplemented vacuity, such as *sháo yào* 芍藥/peony root and *huáng qín* 黄芩/scutellaria root. Inferior medicinal substances are more potent and toxic, and were used to treat specific diseases; they include such herbs as *dà huáng* 大簧/Chinese rhubarb root and *zhì fù zǐ* 炙附子/prepared aconite root. Chinese herbal medicine incorporates the idea of terrain, or *terroir*, at a fundamental level. Medicines come from certain regions where they have been grown and processed by locals for thousands of years, and are then traded as authentic or *dào dì yào cái* 道地藥材 medicinal substances. The classification and production of medicinal substances in China evolved as technology advanced, but the substances always remained intact, linked to their origin and raw form, always resonating with the earth and its material products. Although scholarly labs in China use high-performance liquid chromatography machines and other technologies, the crude form of herbal, mineral, and animal substances has remained a cornerstone of Chinese medicine's connection with nature.

It is a mistake to view Chinese herbal medicine through a biochemical lens—or, rather, we have not developed a sufficiently sophisticated lens through which to evaluate it. For instance, there are many studies that purport to show the "estrogenic" effect of *dāng guī* 当归/Chinese angelica root, and warn of giving it to patients with a history of breast cancer. However, any effect on such patients cannot be evaluated by reactions in a test tube. Pharmacological studies of Chinese medicinal substances must be in the proper context, with respect for the written history of *duì yào* 對藥/herb pairing and formula construction, which has the potential to dramatically alter the effect of any single herb. *Dāng guī* 当归, in itself, is a chemical chameleon; it has tendencies but behaves very differently depending on the other herbs with which it is combined. In other words, Chinese herbs are always seen in relationship to everything else in a formula and to a patient's pattern. All *dāng guī* 当归 is not the same. *Dāng guī* 当归 may be given raw, wine-fried, as a whole root, body only, or just the rootlets (*dāng guī wěi* 当归尾) may be used. Each part of the plant (and its processing) influences the clinical effect. Furthermore, was the plant decocted, made into a tincture, or is it in granule form? What is the dosage? There are only relative situations; Chinese medicine is best when practiced as an art as well as a science. We must practice it ethically and evaluate the risks and benefits via a model that acknowledges the internal safeguards that are part of herbal medicine's history. Chinese medicine is a science of relationships among phenomena and this knowledge base is written in such tomes as the *Shen nong ben cao jing* 神農本草經 and Li Shi-zhen's *Ben cao gang mu* 本草綱目 (*Compendium of Medicinal Herbs*). These works contain the criteria that have been used in the field for centuries, and it is in this context that the safety of polypharmacy as it is used in Chinese medicine has been understood. Chinese herbal medicine is in fact a science with strict rules and protocols for preparing formulas to give to patients; it has a proven safety record.

In contrast, modern pharmaceutical medicine is primarily based on the use of singular, molecular substances that interact with the body in a very direct, forceful way to achieve specific therapeutic effects. In any medical system, the more powerful a specific therapeutic effect, the greater the toxicity and potential for harm. Also, such an approach is one-sided and ignores the inherent complexity of the human organism. Recently a new approach, called combinatorial chemistry, has appeared. This approach uses combinations of drugs to treat various bodily systems, rather than just one targeted organ or tissue. While theoretically this is an advance over the "one drug, one disease" model, and is closer to the clinical reality of patients on multiple medications, no solution has arisen to the increase of drug toxicity that usually occurs when combining many medications. As it stands, it is routine clinical practice to give drugs for side-effects caused by other medications, or for patients with more than one defined disease at any given time.

Biomedicine and Chinese medicine have traditionally been different logical systems, with disparate clinical gazes and diagnostic systems. Whereas biomedicine determines treatment largely on a database of diseases defined by numbers on blood and saliva tests, specific tissue changes, MRIs (magnetic resonance imaging scans), EKGs (electrocardiograms) and so on, Chinese medicine uses other diagnostics (pulse, tongue, abdomen, sensory data, questioning) and a pattern-based approach to treatment that incorporates herbal formulas (rather than single herbs) in its treatments. Herbal formulas, like acupuncture, are complexes that activate the body's innate healing abilities; although exogenous (and allopathic), they affect the endogenous substances of the body. One flaw of biomedicine is that it is often unable to see the rebounding effects of localized treatment with simple drugs or even natural substances to treat disorders. Allopathic medicines are defined as drugs that counter specific symptoms by interfering with natural biological processes, such as using anti-histamines to block histaminic reactions, anticoagulants, antacids, antibiotics. This then shifts pathology to other parts of the bodily terrain. We should expect when we treat symptoms directly with substances such as the single herb *hǎi piāo xiāo* 海螵蛸/cuttlefish bone, which is used in modern China as an antacid, that there will be side-effects as a result, even if they are milder than with medications. It doesn't mean we should altogether avoid allopathic methods, but rather we must be clear about our intentions and motivations as physicians.

One can look at the biomedical technique of HRT (hormone replacement therapy) to see the difference between exogenous substances and endogenous ones, and how they affect the body in substantially different ways. Internally, hormones are produced and controlled by the *yuán qì* 原氣/source qi, which is a combination of *jīng* 精/essence, *gǔ qì* 穀氣/food qi, and *dà qì* 大氣/air qi. They are definitely engendered by *yáng qì* 陽氣, which governs the transformation of all substances of the body. Our bodies are designed to ingest crude substances from nature, such as whole, unrefined foods and medicinal herbs, and our body's process of qi transformation then separates clear yang from turbid yin, and manufactures its vital substances accordingly. With the example of HRT, injecting or ingesting a relatively pure substance—one that is pharmacologically fixed by fractionalizing, as in the case of estrogen and progesterone—reduces the involvement of the qi transformation processes relative to, for example, phytoestrogens from food sources. This problem is the same for all "replacement" therapies, including giving insulin, thyroid, prednisone, and other purified essences that the body would normally synthesize by itself. When the body doesn't need to make its own vital substances, the "side-effect" is that the yang qi is not engaged, and the body becomes flooded with purified essences that can lead to engorgement and yin accumulation (for instance, the side-effects of birth control pills or HRT, including acne, weight gain, and blood circulation problems, specifically, blood stasis due to cold and damp-phlegm accumulation). Side-effects are considered the cost of modern pharmaceutical technologies; Chinese medicine provides a lens through which to evaluate that cost on the body and its new normal or altered physiology.

While the language of biomedical science comes from biology, chemistry, cybernetics, and other scientific disciplines, many of its observations can be related to the systems approach of Chinese medicine. While not based on channel theory and qi, systems biology recognizes that reductionism cannot finally explain the complex interactions between cells, tissues, organs, nerves, other structures, and the communications systems that keep everything functioning in balance. It is here, perhaps, where a mutual understanding of human health and disease between East and West can begin to flourish. If we practice Chinese medicine's technology (needle and moxibustion therapy, herbal medicine) primarily aiming to treat biomedical diseases, and then explain our treatment through biomedical logic, we are essentially practicing a second-rate Western medicine. Rather, we should be true to the foundation of Chinese medicine. How can our tools ever compete with the strength and precision of surgical interventions or the power of drugs? We must practice Chinese medicine according to its essential strengths, as has been done for two thousand years. Ultimately, there is a real zen about the entire process of pulse diagnosis, palpation, questioning, and formulating a treatment plan. The treatment embodies both the practitioner and the patient, and creates a space for healing to occur. It is a gestalt that is greater than the sum of its parts, and both patients and practitioner know when they inhabit this sacred space. Furthermore, just as we study modern medicine and embrace its strengths and note its weaknesses, modern biomedical health professionals should also embrace and study traditional medical systems such as Chinese medicine.

CHAPTER IV

THE PICASSO PRINCIPLE
Developing Multivalent Diagnostic Acumen

医易相同。天人一理也， 一此阴阳也。医道虽繁，而可 一言以蔽之者，曰: 阴阳而已

Medicine and the Yi Jing are the same. [This is because] Nature/heaven and the human body conform to the same laws, namely, the principles of yin-yang. And though medical practice is complicated, we can use yin-yang to summarize and analyze all its permutations.

Zhang Jie-bin, translated by Lifang Qu and Mary Garvey[1]

凡大醫治病，必當安神定志，無欲無求，先發大慈惻隱之心

In all cases, when you treat disease as an eminent physician, you must quiet your shén and fix your intention, you must be free of wants and desires, and you must first develop a heart full of great compassion and empathy.

Sun Si-miao, translated by Sabine Wilms[2]

---

1   Qu and Garvey 2008: 18
2   Sun, S. (S. Wilms trans.) 2012

In *Yi jing's Epistemic Methodology Lifang,* Qu and Mary Garvey discuss a three-part classification system in the *Yi jing* that can be applied to understand fundamental differences between Chinese/Asian medicine and Western biomedicine: *dào* 道/what is above form, *xiàng* 象/image, and *qì* 器/form. "What is above the form is called the *dào* 道."[3] Garvey and Qu define *dào* 道 as the universal potential before space, time and movement. *Xiàng* 象 is defined as a bridge linking the invisible (dào 道) with the visible world (*qì* 器). The *Su wen* speaks in detail about *zàng xiàng* 臟象/visceral manifestation, the ability to see internal processes and structural conditions on the outside of the body. It is central to *zàng xiàng xué* 臟象學/ visceral manifestation theory, which focuses on processes and transformations in the human entity, or what Paul Unschuld calls "systematic correspondence." In contrast, *zàng qì xué* 臟器學/visceral form theory, central to biomedicine, focuses on specific structures and their measurements. In biomedicine, causative factors are seen to be physical, such as morphology, organic changes, and pathogens.

In classical Chinese medicine diagnosis, there are a number of different possible perspectives from which to view your patient. What Michel Foucault, medical anthropologist, called the "clinical gaze",[4] does not have to be limited to one expression. This explains why there are so many different styles of practice in Chinese medicine. Chinese medicine, and its exports to Korea, Japan and Southeast Asia have regional styles and "flavors." This is not an excuse for an anything goes approach; the practitioner cannot just pull a diagnosis out of thin air. It is also not an excuse for throwing everything in the kitchen sink and having too many diagnoses and trying to treat all over the map. There is a fine balance between simplicity and the inherent complexity of the human being. When you look at this complexity of the human being, all of a

3   Qu and Garvey 2008: 19
4   For more information refer to Michel Foucault's (2003) *The Birth of the Clinic*

sudden you can look at it from different angles or perspectives, depending on where you stand. It is all about perspective and all the influences that come in from that relationship between the practitioner and the patient. This involves physiological, emotional, psychological, and spiritual perspectives, sometimes simultaneously.

We have different types of diagnostic "lenses" that we use in Chinese medicine, therefore it is possible to have different diagnoses for the same patient, depending on the training of the practitioner. It is also possible for our diagnosis (as in any form of medicine) to reflect our cognitive and physiological biases. In other words, everyone has a unique constitution which colors their world view. What influences the physician influences his view of the patient, therefore one must develop as non-biased a perspective as possible. In biomedicine, one uses what is believed to be "objective science," based on scans, blood tests, and MRIs to prevent physician bias. But perhaps physical sciences are the result of biases based in a particular world view that underlies biomedicine!

What is often difficult to convey to students of Chinese and Asian medical systems are the different metaphors that inform a pre-modern approach to medicine from the more technological, mechanistic metaphors of modern biomedicine. Chinese medicine speaks in terms of rivers, flows, winds, circular movements, breaths and transformations, rather than in fixed entities that are measured, categorized and prescribed for.[5]

Sun Si-miao says that the *dà yī* 大醫/superior/great physician must practice self-cultivation, centering oneself to calm one's emotions, so as to temper one's own biases. As Chinese medical physicians, we must be aware of how our own constitutions and predispositions may color our diagnosis and treatment. For example, if we are heavy coffee drinkers, it will

---

5   Although both the *Ling shu* and *Nan jing* measure the size of viscera, the length of bowels and acupuncture channels—it is quite incredible considering that these texts were written 2000 years ago

affect our system in such a way that we may not be able to recognize the effects of coffee on speeding up the pulse, or in the demeanor and behavior of our patients! If we are emotionally stressed or imbalanced, we may not be able to be centered enough to concentrate on the fine details of taking the pulse, asking the right questions, or formulating a diagnosis. We also tend to attract patients according to our own physiological or emotional/psychological type, so that if we tend to run to the fatigued or chilly side, we will attract patients who need warm supplementation. As we gain experience and broaden our horizons through study, we will develop more flexibility and be able to mirror our patient's disharmonies correctly without superimposing our own. As it says in the *Su wen*, "shut all of the doors and windows, focusing one's *shén* 神 on the needle."[6]

It is important that a Chinese medical physician lives a lifestyle that personifies the teachings of the medicine, not only using its tools (acupuncture, dietetics, herbal medicine) in clinical practice, but promoting *yǎng shēng* 養生/nourishing life practices. Our diagnostic (and treatment) tools are our minds, hearts, judgement and sense organs, which pick up impressions from our patients and their environment, and we must be as healthy and well rested as possible to perform our work correctly. As Sun Si-miao points out in the quote at the start of this chapter, one must have a mind that is calm and centered, and not focused on desires.

The "Picasso Principle" recognizes that human beings are multi-faceted, and that the physician must make the effort to see the patient as completely as possible. Picasso and other Cubist painters of the early and mid-20th century developed multiple perspectives when looking at the same phenomenon or object in what we call reality. There was a shift from interpreting how the eyes viewed nature, to how the mind sees reality. Just as Picasso used perceptions beyond the standard three dimensions in his Cubist paintings, we can bring in other

---

6   Unschuld and Tessenow 2011: 230

dimensions of diagnosis as a result of the *yuán wù bǐ lèi* 援物
比類 (grasping the cause, making an analogy) discussed in *Su
wen* 76, "When the sages treated a disease, they followed the
pattern and guarded the standards. They drew on facts/causes
and compared the likes/analogies."[7] As expressed by Beijing
acupuncturist Zhang Shijie:

> In acupuncture practice, the eight principles, six couples of
> *jīng luò* 經絡, *zàng fǔ* 臟腑, *wèi qì* 衛氣, *yíng qì* 營氣, *xuè* 血
> and the *sān jiāo* 三焦 are not enough to formulate a pattern
> differentiation (*biàn zhèng* 辨證). We must also use the *yuán
> wù bǐ lèi* 援物比類 principle. This method gives us the
> possibility of recognizing the root of the hundred illnesses
> and of unifying the therapeutic practice.[8]

The various types of pattern differentiation are called *zhěn
duàn* 診斷, but this term is often less rigid than in biomedical
diagnosis. It is a "field and systems" approach, very flexible,
and gives room for the physician to address symptoms
as part of a broad canvas. This in turn leads to treatment
that addresses local symptoms in context of the patient's
constitution, present condition, environment, emotional
state and life circumstances. For this reason, acupuncture/
moxibustion treatments and herbal formulas were complex,
multi-ingredient and expanded and contracted focus
according to foreground (major symptoms) and background
(overall pattern and condition).

The templates in the Han dynasty medical classics have
been adapted over Chinese medicine's long history. For example,
Nan jing 16 delineates a diagnostic method of abdominal
palpation associated with the five phases and *wǔ zàng* 五臟/
five yin viscera at different locations circling the navel. This
in turn served as the template for Japanese physicians such
as Isai Misonou, who developed palpation according to

---

7   Unschuld and Tessenow 2011: 659
8   Rossi 2007: 373

visceral locations in the abdomen. Todo Yoshimasu developed the foundation of abdominal palpation (*Fukushin* 腹診) in Kampo herbal medicine from his research in the *Shang han lun*, and used this as his primary diagnostic method. *Fukushin* 腹診 was further advanced by Bunrei Inaba and Yoshitora (Shukuko) Wakuda by the beginning of the 19th century.

During the Jin/Yuan dynasty period (11th to 13th centuries), the *sì dà jiā* 四大家/four great physicians developed differing approaches to the practice of Chinese/Asian medicine, including Liu Wan-su (He-jian), Li Dong-yuan (Ao), Zhu Dan-xi (Zheng-heng), and Zhang Cong-zheng.[9] During this era, physicians adapted classical *Shang han za bing lun* 傷寒雜病論 formulas to conditions, specific patient populations, political situations, environment, climate and availability of medicinals by modifying the original ingredients. Such physicians as Qian Yi, in the early 12th century, developed special, simplified formulas for children based on the five phases and the *wǔ zàng* 五臟/five yin viscera. Many of these formulas are famous today, including *liù wèi dì huáng wán*/six flavor rehmannia pill, *xiè bái sán*/drain the white powder, *qīng gān wán*/clear the liver pill, and *dǎo chì sǎn*/guide out the red powder. Li Dong-yuan built the core of his herbal system on the main ingredients of *liù jūn zǐ tāng*/four gentlemen decoction, including his famous formula, *bǔ zhōng yì qì tāng*/supplement the middle fortify the qi decoction. Centering his medical philosophy on the spleen and stomach's specific function of qi transformation (raising the *qīng qì* 氣/clear qi, descending the *zhuó qì* 濁氣/turbid qi), he would add ingredients to raise the clear yang (*chái hú* 柴胡/bupleurum, *shēng má* 升麻/cimicifuga, *gé gēn* 葛根/kudzu) and descend turbidity (*qīng pí* 青皮/unripe tangerine peel, *chén pí* 陳皮/tangerine peel, *zé xiè* 澤瀉/alisma) along with ingredients to descend turbid yin (*wú zhū yú* 吳茱萸/evodia).

---

9   Other great physicians that sometimes were included in this status were Zhang Yuan-su and Wang Hao-gu.

Li Dong-yuan felt that it was, in the long term, useless to treat branch symptoms or acute disorders with strong herbal formulas or ingredients, as they must first enter the stomach. If these harsh ingredients (too bitter, cold, acrid or dispersing) damage the spleen and stomach, not only is the physician weakening the patient's constitution, but the harsh ingredients will lose their efficacy over time, or fail to reach their target organs in the body. This is what Li Dong-yuan called "death at the hands of the physician," or supplementing repletion and/or draining vacuity. Instead, he developed modular formulas that contained distinct herbal combinations (like a "source code") and could be combined and recombined depending on symptoms, root and branch, but always promoting *yuán qì* 元氣 and spleen/stomach qi at their core. With their foundations in the *Shang han lun*, Li Dong-yuan's formulas when combined with a proper diet based on grains and vegetables, and an active, simple, emotionally balanced lifestyle could both preserve health and prevent and treat disease.

Chinese medicine provides a clear language of how people get ill, the symptoms that manifest, the location of the disorder, and what the treatment strategies should be. The physician tries to determine how to try to reverse the course of disease by developing sophisticated formulas and acupuncture/moxibustion strategies. So, once we get over the false belief that everything modern is superior to the ideas that came in the past, we can study the medical classics with an open mind and see that our medical ancestors had tremendous wisdom to share, wisdom that has been studied and practiced in every generation up to the present era.

CHAPTER V

THE TECHNICIAN AND THE SCHOLAR-PHYSICIAN

The term philosophy, therefore, describes the entirety of intuitive insight, intellectual knowledge, and all concrete activities associated with the art of nourishing life that the ancient master practitioners engaged in.

Zhang Xi-chun, translated by Heiner Fruehauf[1]

The Chinese medical profession appears to be at a crossroads, one requiring some definition of purpose. Practitioners who want to practice a more open-ended, classically inspired form of Chinese medicine need to develop a vision of what needs to be accomplished. The historical basis of modern Chinese medicine needs to be studied and absorbed, and educational models need to be developed and expanded. If we cannot define what is unique in our field, the tools and technology of our medicine will eventually be subsumed into biomedicine and the underlying principles and theory will be lost.

Although there are many potential bridges of collaboration between Chinese medicine and biomedicine, we need to ask ourselves, do we wish to be technicians, or scholar-physicians?

---

1   Zhang 2009: 3

What do we mean by "scholar-physician?"

Chinese medicine is based largely on scholarship and a literary tradition, with the requirement to study essential classical texts, and quote and debate them. The foundations of Chinese medicine are based on principles (yin-yang, five phases, six channels) that require a philosophical and philological approach to the body of knowledge. Traditionally, a physician-in-training needed to study such texts as the *Su wen* (*Simple Questions*), *Ling shu* (*Divine Pivot*), and *Nan jing* (*Classic of Difficulties*) to understand channel/connecting vessel theory, the *Shang han za bing lun* (*Treatise on Cold Damage and Complex Diseases*) to diagnose progressions of disease parts and practice internal medicine.

In China, the concept of the scholar-physician largely was developed during the 12th century Song dynasty through the encouragement of the emperor Huizhong. Huizong initiated the compilation of classical medical texts, and established printing presses and academies to teach medicine. For the first time, the practice of medicine was elevated to a higher social status, making it more attractive for Confucian scholars who didn't want to be limited to being government officials. Medicine continued to develop during the Jin-Yuan dynasties that followed in the works of the great Jin-Yuan dynasty physicians: Li Dong-yuan, Zhang Zi-he, Liu Wan-su and Zhu Dan-xi. This era was considered to be a "renaissance" in Chinese medicine, so great were the developments of the four schools associated with these men. Under the Mongols, much knowledge was shared across the vast lands of the new empire, and an eclectic approach to knowledge was encouraged.

While the modern era has eroded the ideal of the scholar-physician to some degree in China, the importance of scholarship together with clinical practice has survived relatively intact. In the West, however, where the development of Chinese medicine is largely in an embryonic stage, there is still confusion about what direction we should take, in terms of the role of an acupuncturist in the existing health care systems.

The crossroads of modern medicine and its future

The modern biomedical world has seen huge changes in the last 50 years, as vast institutions of hospital chains, pharmaceutical companies, insurance providers, and research institutions have centralized resources and largely usurped the power once in the hands of doctors. According to Paul Unschuld, medical doctors of the present era have largely had their role reduced to that of technicians, because they have lost control over their sources of information, fees, or decision making. Much of the essential data of biomedicine has been outsourced to the areas of organic chemistry, biology, pharmacology, and physiology, which are separate professions and fields of study. The insurance industry largely determines physician fees, what services will be covered, and for how long. Doctors rely largely on information gained from expensive technological testing apparatus, again reinforced by the insurance industry which demands "definitive" diagnoses, leaving little room for physician judgements based on knowledge and experience.

Many people interested in health provider careers were and are drawn to Chinese medicine as a clear alternative to the present biomedical establishment, in the hope of having a relative degree of independence in day-to-day practice. Most practitioners of Chinese medicine are still independent providers, largely with cash practices, in small offices with relatively low overheads. Some practitioners do work in hospitals, medical clinics and chiropractic offices, usually as limited providers of health care under the auspices of a medical doctor (MD), doctor of osteopathy (DO), or chiropractic doctor (DC). Many practitioners, however, are disappointed by a lack of a clear vision on what we should be: therapists or physicians, primary or secondary care, independent providers or not.

The present-day Chinese medical schools in the West are also struggling with these issues, which are not clearly defined by any means at this point.

Modern medicine has also lost the integrity of the physician-patient relationship to a large extent. Health maintenance organizations (HMOs) and insurance companies often choose the physicians and specialists for patients, determine fees, treatments, timing of visits, and duration of treatment. Physicians have ceded control of their *materia medica* to pharmaceutical companies, who pressure physicians to prescribe their medications and avoid "unproven" treatments such as herbal medicines. Gargantuan legal institutions such as the US Food and Drug Administration (FDA), the American Medical Association (AMA), research foundations, and the HMO/insurance complex render the physician as a highly paid employee of a mega-corporation, unable to control even their own information sources in the medical schools.

What are our choices?

There is great pressure on the Chinese medical field to follow suit, to subsume and integrate into the biomedical world. If this should happen, many of the strengths of Chinese medicine could be threatened, because much of what makes Chinese medicine strong could not easily survive in this environment:

1. Individualization of treatment based on physician judgement.

2. Control of medicines and preparations.

3. Determining compatibility of patients and practitioners.

4. Negotiable fees based on cash practice or profession-based insurance.

5. More time, attention and care given to patients.

6. Traditional diagnostic methods and flexible, creative treatment modalities.

Already there are insurance programs that match acupuncturists/herbalists with patients, approve and review diagnosis and treatment codes, sell herbs to the patients, determine fees and hold the practitioners responsible for large amounts of paperwork that take time away from the patient/practitioner relationship. While I do encourage new graduates to work with other health care providers in both private offices and hospitals, it is also important for us to develop clinical environments that are conducive to the practice of a full spectrum of Chinese medicine. This may also mean we need to develop patient in-care facilities, including hospitals where herbal medicine is used, as in China.

A medicine based on philosophy, not data sets

Chinese medicine is based on study of philosophy and principle, the cornerstone of clinical practice. Chinese medical practitioners are also encouraged to have a broad knowledge of the arts and humanities, so that they may have the greatest possible empathy with their patients. The modern trends in medical studies have moved away from philosophical approaches and the humanities to total immersion in the hard sciences. This trend also colors the training of Chinese medical doctors in China, where studies in Confucian doctrine and philosophy ("the classics") has largely been abandoned. In the West, if one reads the works of Sir William Osler, one can see the emphasis on philosophy and the humanities in medical training less than a century ago.

In conclusion, scholar-physicians embody and live the knowledge that is taught to them. The knowledge base belongs to each individual practitioner, instead of a centralized knowledge source based on data from studies and large institutions. Each practitioner's experience is potentially innovative and creative. The knowledge base is stored in the historical and modern Chinese medical literature, which includes natural philosophy and the clinical case studies of generations of physicians with their prescriptions. In order for us to have a healthy future, we need to recognize the roots of our philosophy and practice, and create environments where we can both cultivate the strengths of our profession, and interact with other medical providers and systems from a position of strength and knowledge.

CHAPTER VI

THERMODYNAMICS AND AUTOIMMUNE DISEASE
Essential Principles of Treatment

Chinese medical theory and autoimmune disease

Recently there has been an alarming increase in autoimmune diseases, ranging from allergies to serious disorders such as multiple sclerosis and scleroderma. Approximately 75 percent of autoimmune diseases occur in women, most frequently during the childbearing years. Biomedical thought suggests that hormones play a role, because some autoimmune illnesses occur more frequently after menopause, others suddenly improve during pregnancy, with flare-ups occurring after delivery, while still others will get worse during pregnancy. Autoimmune diseases also may have a genetic component, but, mysteriously, they can occur in families as different illnesses. For example, a mother may have lupus erythematosus; her daughter, diabetes; her grandmother, rheumatoid arthritis. Research is shedding light on genetic as well as hormonal and environmental risk factors that contribute to the causes of these diseases.

Individually, autoimmune diseases are not very common, with the exception of thyroid disease, diabetes, and systemic lupus erythematosus. However, taken as a whole, they represent the fourth largest cause of disability among women in the United States. However, if we also consider other conditions, such as environmental allergies and Crohn's disease as autoimmune disorders, an even larger number of people are affected.

Chinese medicine can be very helpful in the long-term management of patients with autoimmune diseases, but because of their complexity, long duration, periods of remission and aggravation, their diagnosis and treatment is of necessity more complex than most common complaints. However, many autoimmune diseases were recognized over the long history of Chinese medicine, and several seminal texts developed treatment strategies for such patients. The source texts that may be useful today for treating such diseases include the *Shang han lun*, the *Nan jing*, *Pi wei lun* (*Treatise on the Spleen and Stomach*), and the body of literature known as *Wen bing tiao bian* (*Systematized Identification of Warm Disease*).

According to the *Yi zong jin jian* (*The Golden Mirror of Medicine*) a Qing dynasty text, women's diseases differ from men's in terms of menstrual disorders, vaginal discharge, fertility and child bearing, pregnancy, post-partum, breast and uterine diseases. In chapter 1 of the *Su wen*, a women's life cycles are defined as seven-year cycles of development (menses is said to begin around 14 years of age), whereas male life cycles are eight-year cycles. So, we may find clues here as to why women tend to develop autoimmune diseases more than men. The greater complexity of the female body, plus more fluctuations based on cycles of blood, qi, and yin, may contribute to the development of autoimmune disease.

Chinese medicine classifies diseases in two broad categories:

1. *Wài gǎn* 外感/external contractions, caused by exterior evils such as wind, cold, damp, heat, summer heat, and dryness.

2. *Nèi shāng* 內傷/internal damage caused by emotional excesses and taxation from poor diet, lack of rest, overwork and immoderate sexual activity.

The *Shang han lun* and *Wen bing xue* have developed diagnostic and treatment strategies for external contractions, whereas such texts as the *Pi wei lun*, and the *Jin gui yao lue* (*Prescriptions from the Golden Cabinet*) focus on internal damage disorders. But these two divisions are not arbitrary or exclusive; as Zheng Qin-an points out in his commentary on *Shang han lun*, external contractions, if not resolved in the three yang warps/conformations, will progress to the yin/interior portion of the body, harassing the three yin warps, and become a chronic disease.

The *Pi wei lun* has a pivotal statement on which we can focus quite a bit of attention in trying to understand autoimmune disease from a Chinese medical perspective: "Ministerial fire is the fire of the pericardium developing from the lower burner. It is a foe to the original qi. (This yin) fire and the original qi are irreconcilable to each other. When one is victorious, the other must be the loser."[1]

My explanation of this theory is as follows: the ministerial fire, also known as life gate fire (*mìng mén huǒ* 命門火), is the fire of the lower burner that according to the *Nan jing* resides between the two kidneys. Normally, it is like a pilot light, a level flame that maintains the metabolic heat of the organism. If too low, kidney yang vacuity or dual spleen/kidney yang vacuity may develop, leading to cold and sore lower back and legs, clear, copious urination, and diarrhea with undigested food particles (clear food diarrhea). However, if the ministerial fire is stirred, it rises up, damaging the spleen and stomach and disturbing the heart. The ministerial fire is stimulated by overexertion, overwork, alcohol, smoking, recreational drugs such as cocaine, prescription drugs such as prednisone, excessive sexual activity, loud music, violent movies, and late-night partying. This excessive stirring of ministerial fire eventually consumes the *yuán qì* 原氣/original qi, which is composed of *dà qì* 大氣/air qi from the lungs

---

1   Li and Flaws 2004: 82

combined with *gǔ qì* 穀氣/food qi from the spleen and *jīng* 精/essence from the kidneys to support the organism.

Because the original qi becomes debilitated, and the spleen and stomach are weakened, the clear and the turbid are not properly separated. The *qīng qì* 清氣/clear qi circulates and supports the *wèi qì* 衛氣/defense qi, which cannot properly protect the body's exterior, therefore it "collapses" inwards. The defense qi is yang in nature, therefore warm, and this heat collects internally to produce what Li Dong-yuan calls "*yīn huǒ* 陰火" or yin fire, heat that arises from inside the body. This is an evil, debilitating heat that slowly wastes qi, blood and fluids over time. In addition, the harmonious interaction of the *wèi* 衛/defense and *yíng* 營/construction is lost, leaving the exterior unstable and exposed to attack by external evils. Li Dong-yuan writes in the *Pi wei lun*:

> Consequently, there is no yang qi to sustain the constructive and defensive. As they are unable to withstand wind and cold, cold and heat are generated. All this is due to insufficient qi of the spleen and stomach. However, although they look quite the same, this differs essentially from the pattern of external contraction of wind and cold.[2]

In other words, the body may generate symptoms that look like an external wind/cold attack, but is actually an internal condition caused by vacuity of the spleen and stomach. Rather than relying on prescriptions to release the exterior, we need to supplement the spleen and stomach as a core treatment strategy in treating some cases of seasonal allergies, rhinitis, sinusitis, and repetitive events of the common cold.

This may seem to be a complex theoretical explanation for autoimmune disease, but it does show that Chinese medicine has developed an elegant explanation for the autoimmune process. The *Pi wei lun* has in-depth descriptions of disease processes that resemble such "modern" conditions

---

2   Li and Flaws 2004: 86

as multiple sclerosis and other neurological disorders such as ALS (amyotrophic lateral sclerosis) and Parkinson's disease, along with both acupuncture and herbal medicine strategies for treatment. The core of this approach involves healing the spleen and stomach, specifically the function of separating the clear and turbid, restoring the normal ascending function of the spleen and descending function of the stomach and intestines. It also involves eating a proper diet, called the "qīng 清 dàn 淡" or "clear-bland" diet, based on natural foods with no artificial additives or excessive condiments or flavors, and regulating lifestyle and emotions to emphasize peace and equanimity in one's life.

> In this world there are two times. There is mechanical time and there is body time. The first is as rigid and metallic as a massive pendulum of iron that swings back and forth, back and forth, back and forth. The second squirms and wriggles like a bluefish in a bay. The first is unyielding, predetermined. The second makes up its mind as it goes along.[3]

The Nan jing is in essence a meditation on the relationship of human beings to the phenomenon of time, specifically "body time." Several chapters or "difficulties" in the Nan jing are about the relationship of the breath to the pulse, and systematic correspondences between color, sound, odor and palpable sensations. These phenomena are the external manifestations of channel and visceral relationships that not only give us a real-time picture of various illnesses, but also their origin and possible course of development.

The ideal pulse, or movement in the vessels, is perfectly balanced, smooth, pliable and flexible, with an even, moderate rhythm. Beginning from this measurement, variations in speed, quality (rough, fine, soggy), depth, and position (inch, bar and cubit lengthwise, heaven, human and earth depth-wise) show us deviation from this ideal equilibrium. The more complex

---

3   Lightman 2004: 23–24

the disease pattern, the more complex the pulse will be. However, just as in any mathematical computation, we begin from the simplicity of yin and yang qualities into complexity, which are simply variations of yin and yang multiplied by the number of disease factors present. We then determine treatment by synthesizing information from the pulse along with other sensory data and the results of our questioning the patient.

All variations from the norm are called *xié qì* 邪氣/evil qi. *Zhèng qì* 正氣/correct (right) qi is that which maintains normal health and visceral function of the body. Through the pulse and other diagnoses, we try to calibrate the degree, speed, and direction of evil qi versus the ability of correct qi to resist it. Evil qi can include visiting evils, such as wind, cold, damp, heat, summer heat, or dryness, epidemic evils such as damp, warmth and warm toxin disease, or internal evils caused by excessive emotions damaging the viscera and bowels. To support correct qi, we use supplementation or harmonization methods. To attack evil qi, we use sweating, precipitation and purging, vomiting, urination, dispersing and warming. In addition, we may use dietetics, lifestyle modifications, behavioral therapies or meditation and prayer to help strengthen correct qi and eliminate evils. Every disease has to be differentiated by pattern and stage, using the pulse and symptom picture to determine the degree of repletion or vacuity, interior or exterior, heat or cold, location in qi, blood or fluids. We can also determine the stage of the illness using the *liù jīng biàn zhèng* 六經辨證/six channel pattern differentiation from the *Shang han lun*, or the *sì fēn biàn zhèng* 四分辨證/four aspects pattern differentiation of warm disease theory. These systems, or "immunological maps," determine the location, direction of movement, and speed of the evil qi through the channel system, and determine the strength of the correct qi and its ability to resist the evil qi. Warm disease theory also talks about latent evils that have "incubated" deep inside the body from season to season or even over a period of several years.

Once we have determined the location, strength, duration, and direction of the autoimmune disorder, we need to develop long-term treatment strategies in order to "change the direction" of the disease. In other words, we need to direct the disease outwards and away from the yin interior towards the yang exterior to prevent the disease from lodging itself in the blood, fluids or yin viscera. According to Chinese medicine, diseases have "exit routes" through the yang channels and their associated bowels, and most treatment strategies are designed to take advantage of these exit routes, as diseases cannot directly exit from the yin viscera, blood or fluids. Many patients with autoimmune diseases also have weakened, damaged or exhausted *jīng* 精/essence, which can take years of treatment to reverse. Emotional traumas such as death of a loved one, divorce, loss of job, or sudden change in climate or residence can also tax the essence and correct qi, and can contribute to the development of a chronic disease.

For those patients who have a long history of an autoimmune disease, it is very important to take a detailed history, as such diseases as lupus and rheumatoid arthritis often go through several stages of aggravation and remission, with different symptom patterns manifesting at each stage. The experienced practitioner will not rely just on one method of pattern differentiation, but will use what is appropriate, whether it is spleen-stomach theory, five phases, six channel, four aspect, or some combination thereof. The effects of previous or concurrent treatments must also be factored in. Many autoimmune diseases are treated with powerful drugs such as steroids, antibiotics, anti-inflammatories or chemotherapy drugs, and this can alter the symptom picture somewhat, or weaken the correct qi and essence. One then alters treatment accordingly, being cautious about potential drug-herb interactions, and then primarily supporting the correct qi. For example, a patient with later-stage nephrotic syndrome or chronic nephritis may be taking toxic medications to control proteinuria or high creatinine counts, with many side-effects or complications. In such cases, the safest course is to use such herbs as *dōng chóng xià cǎo* 冬蟲夏草/cordyceps, which supplements and protects the kidneys against further damage.

Chronic diseases transform according to natural cycles, such as seasonal changes. They transform, aggravate, worsen, or move towards remission. When the correct qi is strengthened to the point where it can keep the disease in check, this leads to a more optimum level of functionality and stability. It is possible to help our patients with autoimmune diseases return to a more healthy, normal life with Chinese medicine, but we need to be very detailed and observant in our diagnosis and treatment strategies.

Understanding Chinese medicine thermodynamics and autoimmune disease

In my opinion, based on my research into the *Su wen*, the symptoms of autoimmune issues are a result of two major factors: 1) disharmony of *wèi qì* 衛氣 and *yáng qì* 陽氣 and 2) disturbance of the body's ministerial fire distribution, what I call "thermodynamics." Regulating ministerial fire is a major part of how the *Shang han lun* and *Jin gui yao lue* choose formulas to treat associated patterns, specifically *shào yáng* 少陽, *shào yīn* 少陰 and *jué yīn* 厥陰.

The *yáng qì* 陽氣 rises with the sun, and with it, the *wèi qì* 衛氣/defense qi rises to the surface to circulate, following the breath, 25 times during the day, then as the sun sets, the defense qi "sinks" deep into the yin portion of the body (fluids, blood, yin viscera), to rest there. The warmth circulates on the surface and maintains body temperature, regulating the pores and enabling the moistening of the skin and peripheral areas of the body. At night time, according to the *Nan jing*, it rests and regenerates the internal yin viscera. However, if the *wèi qì* 衛氣/defense qi is weak or not harmonized with the *yíng* qì 營氣/construction qi, it may float, and heat will leak out of the pores, leading to sweating, hot flashes, and loss of vitality.

How the *Shang han lun* views cold damage and wind strike as disruption of the body's ministerial fire and yang qi

To understand the deeper essence of the *Shang han lun*, one needs to look at the concept of *shang han* 傷寒/cold damage, which begins with an exterior evil being introduced to the tài yáng 太陽 channel. *Qì huà* 氣化/qi transformation begins much like how the sun rises from the water, moving up and out toward the surface. This process of *qì huà* 氣化/ qi transformation lies at the heart of the *Shang han lun*. At the exterior, water vapor is expelled from the skin and pores, and at the interior, water is expelled through the urinary ducts. Water at the surface is like mist or fog; and the interior is heavy and turbid like a drainage ditch. If the *tài yáng* 太陽 channel is unimpaired, there are no avenues for *xié qì* 邪氣/ evil qi to enter the body. When *tài yáng* 太陽's *qì huà* 氣化/ qi transformation is weakened or impaired, *xié qì* 邪氣/evil qi invades and blocks the pores, leading to *shāng hán* 傷寒/cold damage, whatever the time of day or season.

In the early stages, the evil is relatively weak and the *zhèng qì* 正氣/correct qi still has strength. If diagnosed correctly, the *xié qì* 邪氣/evil qi can be dispelled and *zhèng qì* 正氣/ correct qi will recover. If incorrectly diagnosed and treated, the *zhèng qì* 正氣/correct qi will be weakened and the *xié qì* 邪氣/ evil qi will be strengthened. The illness then will grow deeper and transform from channel to channel, bowel to bowel, eventually leading to *hé bìng* 合病/combination diseases of multiple channels. Once it reaches the *jué yīn* 厥陰 stage, with it's roots intact, it may re-emerge at the *tài yáng* 太陽 over time, causing various complex disease to develop, eventually leading to a separation of yin and yang, and various life-threatening diseases.

Zheng Qin-an says that the nature of *shāng hán* 傷寒/ cold damage is in the dynamics of the *tài yáng* 太陽, not necessarily the exterior evil itself. It is the effect on *qì huà* 氣化/qi transformation, not the evil, which can be cold, hot, damp, and so on. More importantly, it sets the stage for the development of our *nèi shāng* 內傷/internal damage and autoimmune issues later on.[4]

---

4   For more information on the work of Zheng Qin-an refer to Dr. Yaron Seidman's Zheng Qin-an Project at http://hunyuan.org/index.html

CHAPTER VII

MÀI XIÀNG 脈象/
PULSE IMAGE
The Core of Chinese
Medical Diagnosis

Perhaps the most precious diagnostic tool of Chinese medicine is pulse diagnosis, and what is called *mài xiàng* 脈象/pulse image or *mài zhěn* 脈診/pulse examination in classical sources.[1] Dr. Mistry, an Ayurvedic physician, explained that "pulse reading is like Zen...through pulse, we reconstruct the entire chain of events, the entire etiology of the illness, from first cause to immediate complaint."[2] What is unique about the pulse, or "movement in the vessels" model as Paul Unschuld translates it, is that it is both holographic and local, rooted in real time but acknowledging the history of the patient's condition in the past (*bìng yīn* 病因/disease origin or etiology), and future (*yù hòu* 預後/prognosis). Pulse diagnosis is also related architecturally to different parts of the body, based on proportions in a small region at the wrist, divided into three sections (*cùn* 寸/inch, *guān* 關/gate, and *chǐ* 尺/foot), three depths (*tiān* 天/heaven, *rén* 人/humanity, and *dì* 地/earth), length, width, depth, fullness, emptiness, speed, direction, order/chaos. In the interests of space, and the focus

---

1   Note that *zàng xiàng* 臟象/visceral manifestation also contains the notion of *xiàng* 象/imagery

2   Langford 1999: 42

of what I am trying to present in this book, we are going to focus on what Elisabeth Hsu calls the *cùn* 寸/inch, *guān* 關/gate, *chǐ* 尺/foot pulse model, established in the *Nan jing* as the definitive text in historically describing this model. Within this model, later physicians, especially during the Song/Jin/Yuan dynasties, made minor variances, and these are also included in Appendix IV. According to Elisabeth Hsu, "neither the *Su wen* or *Ling shu* mention the *cùn* 寸/*guān* 關/*chǐ* 尺 method, while the *Mai jing* (*Pulse Classic*) and *Nan jing* discuss it quite extensively. The medieval Dunhuang manuscript texts, in particular, accord this method foremost importance."[3] The excavations that are ongoing in the Dunhuang caves show a remarkable convergence of medical traditions between Chinese, Tibetan, Indian and Greco-Arabic physicians in this remote desert oasis.

The *Su wen*, *Ling shu* and *Nan jing* developed pulse models that conformed to the Han dynasty philosophers' views of the natural world. They were based on:

- five directions (north, south, east, west and center)

- five seasonal qi influencing the pulse (winter, spring, summer, long summer, autumn)

- three positions corresponding to the three burners (upper, middle and lower) and three depths corresponding to heaven, humanity and earth

- five seasonal pulse qualities (*gōu* 鈎/hook-like, *máo* 毛/hair-like, *xiàn* 線/wiry, *huǎn* 緩/leisurely/moderate, and *shí* 石/sinking/stone-like

- 28 pulse qualities associated with disease patterns

- dimensional/architectural relationships of 12 channel positions in six wrist positions.

---

3   Hsu 2008: 2

These dimensional/architectural relationships were based on the *jīng mài* 經脈/channel/vessel system, that visualized a system of channels that began in the upper and lower limbs, flowing to and from fingertips and toes, and penetrating the interior of the body, according to a three-yin/three-yang schematic. It was designed as a methodology and map for viewing spacial, causal relationships of the interior and exterior, viscera and bowels, qi, blood and fluids.

Various pulse schemata included additional layers of the *jīng mài* 經脈 system, such as the *qí jīng bā mài* 奇經八脈/ eight extraordinary vessels, which are the "energetic" blueprint for the physical body,[4] the *luò mài* 絡脈/network vessels, and the *bié mài* 別脈/divergent vessels that connect with the *zàng fǔ* 臟腑/viscera and bowels. The pulse maps were designed to interpret this physiological domain, and the physician responds by treatment with acupuncture, moxibustion, and internal/herbal medicine.

Pulse influences

When heaven and earth are warm and harmonious, then the main waters are quiet and calm. When heaven is cold and the earth is frozen, then the main waters congeal so that [their flow] is impeded. When heaven has summer heat and the earth is hot, then the main waters [gush forth as if] boiling and overflow. When a sudden wind rises violently, then the main waters gush up in breakers and rise [like] ridges [in the fields]. Now, when evil enters the vessels, if it is cold, then the blood congeals so that [its flow] is impeded. If it is summer heat, then the qi is saturated with moisture. When subsequently a depletion evil enters [the vessels] and settles [there], then this, too, is similar to when the main waters are affected by wind: The arrival of the vessel movement in the

---

4　See Yoshio Manaka's discussion of the extraordinary vessels in chapter 5 of *Chasing the Dragon's Tail* (1995)

conduits, at times it, too, rises [like] the ridges [in the fields]. Its passage in the vessels is continuous. (*Su wen* 27, Discourse on the Division and Union of True and Evil Qi)[5]

Over different eras in the history of Chinese medicine, different pulse systems and schema were developed, associated with different medical currents: *Shang han lun* (*liù jīng* 六經/six warps/conformations), *Su wen*, *Ling shu*, *Nan jing*, *Mai jing* (Wang Shu-he) and physicians of the Jin-Yuan, Song and Ming dynasties (such as Zhang Jing-yue, Liu Wan-su, and Li Dong-yuan).[6] They reflected the interests of the physicians who lived in various epochs of Chinese history, from the Han to the Qing dynasty, according to the prevalence of different illnesses in the societies in which these physicians lived. These models can give us inspiration and focus in 21st-century practice, with the often unusual and complex patterns that we see in post-modern patients. Many modern practitioners become confused by these different models, not realizing that they are representational models of acupuncture channels and visceral systems designed to allow a physician to focus on the essential information and develop one's own pulse vocabulary. Over years of observing patients, I've seen conditions that did not fit into strictly traditional categories, and had to identify pulse qualities that required new interpretations in new contexts. The most significant change in the modern era has been patients using multiple medical systems, medications, supplements, and recreational drugs (along with exposure to environmental toxins such as radiation and pesticides). Add to this transcontinental travel with routine crossing of time zones at high speeds, and a new range of influences on people's health and their pulses requires even deeper insight on the part of the Chinese medical physician.

---

5   Unschuld and Tessenow 2011: 448–449
6   See Appendix IV for these pulse maps

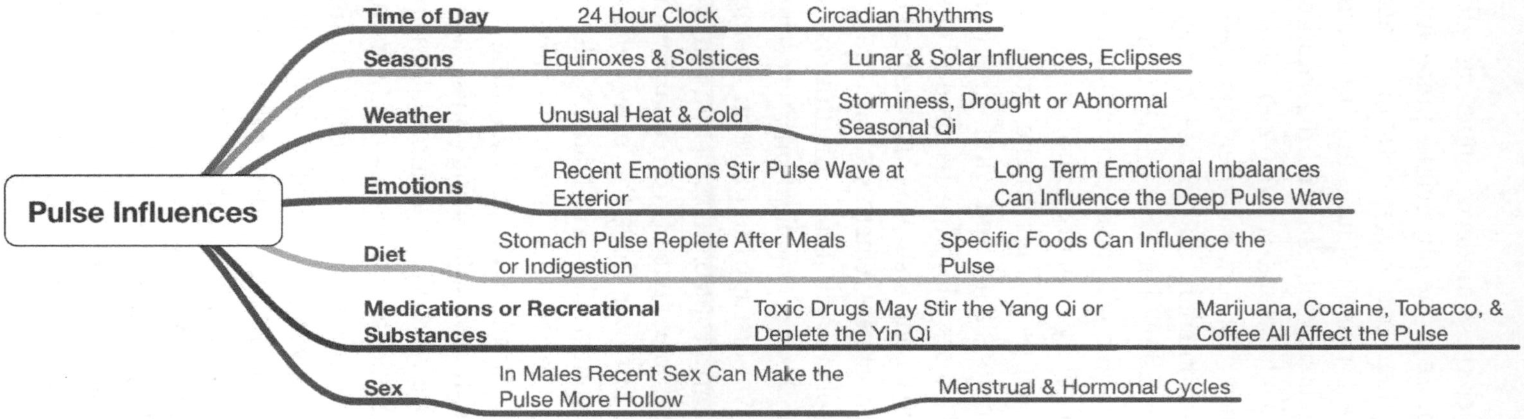

Figure 7.1: *Pulse influences*

Pulse Influences

Time of Day — 24 Hour Clock — Circadian Rhythms

Seasons — Equinoxes & Solstices — Lunar & Solar Influences, Eclipses

Weather — Unusual Heat & Cold — Storminess, Drought or Abnormal Seasonal Qi

Emotions — Recent Emotions Stir Pulse Wave at Exterior — Long Term Emotional Imbalances Can Influence the Deep Pulse Wave

Diet — Stomach Pulse Replete After Meals or Indigestion — Specific Foods Can Influence the Pulse

Medications or Recreational Substances — Toxic Drugs May Stir the Yang Qi or Deplete the Yin Qi — Marijuana, Cocaine, Tobacco, & Coffee All Affect the Pulse

Sex — In Males Recent Sex Can Make the Pulse More Hollow — Menstrual & Hormonal Cycles

Figure 7.1 outlines these modern influences, all of which are potential disruptors of the physician's pulse analysis. Tibetan physicians tell their patients not to have sexual relations the night before a pulse reading, and to avoid alcohol and spicy, greasy foods as well, as taxed digestion can produce a slippery pulse, while sexual activity can cause a hollowness in the male pulse. Unusual weather changes, including the present-day phenomenon of climate change, will always affect the pulse reading. For example, here in San Diego the late summer monsoon will raise the humidity and heat levels, and I find most of my patients manifesting a floating, rapid and soggy pulse on those days. In the autumn, desert winds blow in (the famous "Santa Ana wind" phenomenon), drying out the air, and pulses will often become flooding and rapid on these occasions. Long-distance travel, especially to areas in the southern hemisphere, where seasons are opposite to the northern hemisphere, can cause disruption of the normal seasonal pulses. Use of medications, especially the more powerful ones, will disrupt the pulse in dramatic ways. For example, use of birth control pills, high in estrogen, will create a pulse that resembles that of a pregnant woman; in other words, slippery. But over time, the heavy, damp, stagnating nature of birth control pills will lead to cold, phlegm/damp accumulation in the abdomen, and in turn cold blood stasis, which will slowly "strangle" the pulse, leading to a more sè 澀/ choppy, and eventually "suffocating" pulse (where the vessel becomes harder to read due to accumulations of static blood and phlegm). Emotional upsets can range from heavy traffic on the way to an appointment, to deep traumas suffered by emotional abuse, divorce, death of a close relative, friend or spouse, or loss of a job. All of these can create "ripples" that can be read in the pulse, due to their destabilizing influences. But all of these phenomena can be included and explained both in terms of their influence on the pulse, and the patterns of the patient as well. See Appendix I: Drugs and their Effects on the Pulse for more information.

Nan jing pulse diagnosis

In the *Nan jing*, every illness is viewed through timing, direction, and manifestation. In diagnosing your patient, you first have to determine the *zhèng cháng mài* 正常脈/normal pulse, taking into account the season, the constitution of the patient, emotional factors, diet, and medications. Once the normal pulse has been determined, the physician can then determine *xié qì* 邪氣/evil qi in its various forms; *wài gǎn* 外感/exterior contractions such as wind, cold, damp, dryness, or heat; *nèi shāng* 內傷/internal damage by emotions, food, taxation or visceral disharmonies. For external contractions, we may use *liù jīng biàn zhèng* 六經辨證/six channel differentiation, for internal damages, *wǔ xíng xué shuō* 五行學說/five phase theory or *zàng fǔ xué shuō* 臟腑學說/viscera-bowel theory. There are basically two categories of medical strategies. The first is *gōng xié* 攻邪/attacking (disease) evils, especially when there are replete qi in the body; the second is *fú zhù zhèng qì* 扶助正氣/supporting the correct qi. Sometimes the evil must be removed forcefully, without damaging the correct qi, and sometimes the correct qi must be strengthened, which can then overcome and repel or absorb the evil on its own. The correct strategy will depend on timing, the speed of the disease (aggressive, yang and swift, or weak, yin and slow), and the stage of the disease. This is where *Shang han lun* six-channel differentiation becomes essential; one can then determine where in the course of an externally contracted illness the patient is "staging the battle". With internal disharmonies, it may be a matter of harmonizing five-phase relationships of viscera and bowels.

One needs to draw a map of the *bìng yīn* 病因/disease origin, how long ago in time, and where on the timeline the disease is manifesting. Is it in the (yang) channel stage? Has it entered the tissues associated with the five yin viscera? Or has it penetrated the yin portion of the body, which means that very sophisticated strategies of supplementation and drainage must be applied?

The pulse system that I've relied on in my clinical practice for the past 35 years is based on the one described in *Nan jing*, chapters 1–23. I have found it to be flexible in describing both channel/vessel conditions for acupuncture/moxibustion, and the contents of the *sān jiāo* 三焦/triple burner for internal medicine. I will discuss here three of the most significant chapters that are most essential to the practice of pulse diagnosis.

Nan jing 1: Origin of the pulse system

The *cùn kǒu* 寸口/inch-opening constitutes the *huì xué* 會穴/great meeting point of the contents passing through the vessels; it is the section of the hand *tài yīn* 太陰 channel where the movement in that vessel can be felt.[7]

When a normal person inhales once, the content of the vessels proceeds three *cùn* 寸/(body) inches; when a normal person exhales once, the contents also proceed three (body) inches. Exhaling and inhaling constitutes one breathing period. During this period, the contents of the vessels proceed six inches. A person, in the course of one day and night (24 hours), breathes altogether 13,500 times. During this time, the contents of the vessels proceed through 50 passages. The *wèi qì* 衛氣/defense qi and *yíng qì* 營氣/construction qi proceed through 25 passages during a yang period, and through 25 passages during a yin period. This constitutes one cycle. Because the contents of the vessels meet again, after 50 passages, with the inch opening, this section is the beginning and the end of the movement of the content of the vessels through the body's five yin viscera and six bowels. Hence, the pattern (of death or life, good or evil auspices harbored by the five yin viscera and six bowels) is obtained from the inch opening.[8]

7   Unschuld 2016 (*Nan jing*): 49
8   Unschuld 2016 (*Nan jing*): 49–50

Much of significance can be obtained from a close reading of
Nan jing 1:

- The relationship of movement in the vessels and
  breathing rhythms.

- The relationship of defense qi and construction qi to
  their circulation with the contents of the vessels.

- A standard for the normal pulse, out of which deviations
  to equilibrium and health can be obtained.

- The movements of the vessel contents between yang
  phases (daytime) and yin phases (nighttime).

To this, in later chapters, the *Nan jing* adds seasonal qualities to
the pulse (*Nan jing* 18), and six-paired channel qualities to the
pulse (in *Nan jing* 7, also associated with seasonal qi).

Nan jing 15: Seasonal correspondences of pulses

> In spring the movement in the vessels is *xiàn* 線/wiry/
> string-like, in summer *gōu* 鉤/hook-like; in autumn *máo* 毛/
> hair-like; in winter, *shí* 石/stone-like. These movements are in
> accordance with the four seasons.[9]

Each season has it's own particular *qì* 氣 characteristic that
expresses itself in the vessel flow. Winter is the time of *yīn
qì* 陰氣, so the pulse is sinking like a stone, heavy and deep,
like hibernating insects. Spring is the time of the return of life,
when the qi rises to the surface, and tries to break through the
limitations of the remaining yin/cold, so it is *xiàn* 線/tense/
wiry. In summer, the *yáng qì* 陽氣 movement is completely
uninhibited, like rushing mountain streams, so the pulse floods
outwards. Because the yang movement is strong, and the yin
(sinking) movement is weak, the movement in the vessels

---

9   Unschuld 2016 (*Nan jing*): 49

under the fingers feels like a *gōu* 鉤/hook. In late summer, a transitory period of equilibrium is reached, and the earth (*tài yīn* 太陰) phase predominates, so a balanced, *huǎn* 緩 relaxed/moderate movement is felt. In the autumn, an inward, contracting movement has begun, but because much of the *yáng qì* 陽氣 has been spent and scattered through outward expression, such as sweating and exertion, the pulse is soft, fine, and just under the skin. According to the *Su wen*, any abnormal expression in the pulse that does not match the season means either a disharmony between the person and the season/environment, or the seasons are not expressing themselves in the proper order. In Chinese medicine, this is expressed as *zhǔ qì* 主氣/host qi and *kè qì* 客氣/guest qi, the normal season being the host, the abnormal season being the guest. In other words, if the winter lasts too long into springtime, we say the *kè qì* 客氣/guest qi (winter) has overwhelmed the *zhǔ qì* 主氣/host qi (spring).

Each seasonal pulse quality can be overly strong and replete, indicating illness, in the yang section/exterior of the body. The pulse can also be vacuous in its seasonal quality, indicating illness in the yin portion/interior of the body. The text goes on to describe other abnormal qualities of the seasonal pulses, indicating different severities of disease.

In addition, a healthy seasonal pulse is always seen to contain stomach qi, associated with earth. The earth quality, described as *huǎn* 緩/relaxed and moderate, should be felt in all of the seasonal pulses as a suppleness and pliability in the vessel. For the spring *xiàn* 線/tense/wiry pulse, it would feel wiry but flexible, like fresh green branches, whereas a lack of stomach qi would feel hard and brittle, like dead branches.

Nan jing 16: Correspondences of emotion, complexion and symptoms with pulse images

Any verification of a disease should be based on the presence of certain internal and external evidence. For example, consider feeling a pulse (movement in the vessels) that is associated with a disease in the liver.

> External evidence of such a disease includes a tendency towards tidy appearance, a virid face, and an inclination to become angry. Internal evidence of such a disease is the presence of *dòng qì* 動氣/stirring qi to the left of the navel which, if pressed, response with firmness and pain. The disease, as perceived by the patient, consists of four swollen limbs, closure and protuberance illness, difficult urination and defecation, as well as twisted muscles. If this evidence is present, the liver is afflicted.[10]

Nan jing 16 emphasizes that pulses are combined with other diagnostic criteria, such as viewing the complexion, emotional qualities, and abdominal palpation. Each five-phase pulse, associated with one of the yin viscera, needs to be confirmed by symptoms, emotions, questioning, complexion, and abdominal palpation. However, the most complex diagnostic system available to us is the pulse/movement in the vessels, as a non-verbal, non-biased method for reading real-time disharmonies in our patients. All of the other methods are generally confirmatory, as diagnostic and treatment strategies both in the acupuncture classics and herbal classics are firmly based on the pulse.

---

10 Unschuld 2016 (*Nan jing*): 184–185

Nan Jing 18: Establishing the pulse positions and their associated qualities

Nan jing 18 unites two systems and their 'maps' of pulse diagnosis:

1. The diagnosis of the *zàng fǔ* 臟腑/viscera/bowels, located according to their position from above to below, from heaven position to earth position.

2. The circulation of the 12 primary (acupuncture) channels, through the medium of five-phase theory, according to the "circular theory of classical Chinese medicine."

This model places fire at the top (southerly direction), water at the bottom (northerly direction), wood east, and metal west, with earth at the center. There are two physiological "fires," *jūn huǒ* 君火/sovereign fire associated with the heart (above), *xiàng huǒ* 相火/ministerial fire associated with the *mìng mén* 命門/life gate and kidney (below). The *xīn zhǔ* 心主/heart governor and *sān jiāo* 三焦/triple burner are associated with *xiàng huǒ* 相火/ministerial fire, which circulates in the *shào yáng* 少陽 and *jué yīn* 厥陰 channels and domains. In some pulse systems, they are palpated in the third/foot position on the right wrist. In other systems, they are associated with the "right kidney," or "kidney yang," which is basically expressing the same concept. In *Nan jing* 18, the *jūn huǒ* 君火/sovereign fire is represented on the *cùn* 寸/inch position on the left wrist, which sinks to and connects with the *chǐ* 尺/foot position on the right wrist where the *xiàng huǒ* 相火/ministerial fire is represented (see diagram in Appendix VI: *Nan jing* 18 Pulse Model).

The first criteria that must be established by the physician is what we can call the "normal pulse." This is the constitutional pulse that must be calculated for each patient.

It is like this. The three sections concerned are inch, gate and foot. The nine indicator levels refer to surface, center and depth (of each section). The upper section is patterned on heaven; it is governed by illnesses located from the chest upward to the head. The central section is patterned after man; it is governed by illnesses located below the diaphragm to the navel. The lower section is patterned after earth; it is governed by illnesses located below the navel to the feet. Before treatment, first carefully examine the vessels and only then apply the needles. (*Nan jing* 18)[11]

Pulse architecture: a multi-dimensional model

If we look visually at the *cùn kǒu* 寸口/inch-mouth region near the wrist where we primarily read the pulse, we find these parameters, in addition to the nine indicators, three positions and three depths we have previously discussed:

A. Exterior/*zhōng*/center/depth

B. Skin/qi/blood/*zàng fǔ*/bone

C. Five tissues

D. Five levels (*Nan jing* 5: lung/heart/spleen/liver/kidney)

E. Width: short/crowded, long

F. Shape

G. Speed

H. Direction

I. Clarity: thickness, murkiness.

---

11 Unschuld 2016 (*Nan jing*): 206

In the Nan jing pulse system, one begins by reading the *zhèng qì* 正氣 aspect of the pulse, and then measures the *xié qì* 邪氣 in relationship to this. One uses the parameters of a balanced pulse wave, modified by the constitution of the patient, season, and location (climate and environmental conditions). Once we have determined this, we can read the deviation from the *zhèng qì* 正氣 correct state to determine the *xié qì* 邪氣/evil qi aspect. For example, a recent strong emotional upset can scatter the pulse (*sǎn mài* 散脈), *zhòng fēng* 中風/wind strike will cause the pulse to float, stagnant bowels will causing a sinking, firm/tense pulse. The more complex the disorder, the more combinations of pulse qualities will be evident in the reading. For example, in patients with complex, long-term conditions such as cancer, and autoimmune disorders such as lupus or rheumatoid arthritis, I will often feel what I call a "humoral" pulse, which feels like several strands of movement wrapping around each other like coiled worms or snakes. In such situations, complex and multiple interventions may be necessary to restore a sense of equilibrium and give the *zhèng qì* 正氣 the upper hand, including acupuncture/moxibustion, herbal medicine, diet, exercises, and lifestyle changes.

In concluding this condensed, but hardly exhaustive pulse section of the book, I am of necessity not including pulse references and materials from the *Mai jing* 脈經, *Shang han lun* 傷寒論, *Jin gui yao lue* 金匱要略, *Bin hu mai xue* 瀕湖脈學, and other sources that should be a focus of study for the classical Chinese medicine practitioner. The purpose of this book is to "boil down" the classical teachings of medicine to their essence. Perhaps at a later time, this will all be part of a broader book devoted to the subject of pulse diagnosis.

NARRATIVE (Z'ev Rosenberg interview, May 2017)

In terms of teaching pulse diagnosis, you have a number of problems. The first is that people teaching in our Western Chinese medicine schools largely don't have enough pulse skills themselves to inspire confidence in the students. There is a process to teaching pulses and transmission, it's not just studying the techniques, it's also confirming and working with a teacher, and when you practice acupuncture seeing how the pulses change before, after, and during a treatment. You need all this confirmation, and there are many practitioners who say that pulse diagnosis isn't important, it's too subjective. It is not a good outcome if practitioners are made to feel embarrassed about using these "primitive" methods in this era of technological medicine and diagnostic devices. However, using machines to diagnose has its own limitations, and while many of these machines such as EKGs and MRIs can be very useful, all technology is merely the application of medical philosophies and their views of the human entity. This is both a benefit and limitation. Pulse diagnosis allows the physician to have a direct, real-time connection with a patient, and at the same time gain a great deal of complex, essential information about the patient's health.

Many years ago, I had the honor to study not only with Chinese doctors, but also with Tibetan and Ayurveda physicians. When I was in acupuncture college, it had three departments: Chinese medicine, Ayurvedic medicine and body therapies. A small part of my training was with Dr. Vasant Lad, who today is the head of the Ayurvedic Institute in Albuquerque.

He said, "When you are feeling the pulse you are feeling the life of the patient in your hands." You are feeling the pulse of life, it's something moving and changing, holographic in that it deals with the entire condition of the patient in real time. We divide the pulse into three parts, *cùn* 寸/inch, *guān* 關/gate, and *chǐ* 尺/foot, upper, middle lower burner and the three depths, *tiān* 天/heaven, *rén* 人/humanity, and *dì* 地/earth. It's a holographic grid to view the overall condition of the patient and according to the maps in the Chinese medical classics, specifically the *Su wen* and the *Nan jing*. It's our primary diagnostic tool! Ironically in my early days of study and practice it was difficult to find Chinese practitioners who really emphasized the pulse, because modern TCM largely ignored or over-simplified it to correspond with modern medical diagnosis. But soon after I graduated TCM school, I moved to Colorado and took a seminar with Dr. Yeshi Dhonden, physician to the Dalai Lama, who didn't speak English but felt my pulses and told me exactly what was going on with my health. Some years later, another Tibetan physician (Dr. Lobsang Ropgay) came to San Diego and did a presentation through UC San Diego Medical School with 18 cancer patients. He felt their pulses and without asking any questions he was able to tell 17 out of 18 patients what type of cancer they had from the pulse. To the 18th patient he said, "You don't have cancer," and he was correct on all of his diagnoses. It was a powerful demonstration of what the potential of pulse diagnosis can be.

My policy is when I have a new patient, I don't let them tell me what's going on first. I feel the pulse, look at the tongue, and do the visual diagnosis. The value of that is twofold: 1) You reframe the condition the patient has, in other words you already bring the person's condition and the patient themselves into the context of which you work and that's very important; and 2) We are not trying to duplicate Western medicine, though there are many practitioners who feel they should. It's very difficult to treat Western diseases as a separate entity from a Chinese medical lens. You reframe it and feed back to the person through the pulse what's going on with them, not just physiologically, but emotionally, psychologically and even spiritually. One of the traditional roles of the physician is to give meaning to the patient's suffering, and a direction for them to take to truly relieve that suffering. And as you reflect this back to them, it builds patient confidence, and it is better than any practice-building seminar, one could hope to take. The word of mouth from such diagnosis can only spread and build your practice.

CHAPTER VIII

ZÀNG XIÀNG 藏象/ VISCERAL MANIFESTATION
The Core of Chinese Medical Diagnostic Systems

The five long-term depots, with them [man] corresponds to heaven and earth. They are associated with [the dynamics of] yin and yang [qi]. They correspond to the four seasons and they are transformed in accordance with the five sections [of the five phases]. Among the five long-term depots there are small and big ones, those located above and others located below. Those that are hard and others that are brittle, those that stand upright and others that are inclined.

(*Ling shu* 47)[1]

Su wen and *Ling shu* have multiple chapters discussing fractal relationships, including *Ling shu* 46 (The Five Modifications) and *Ling shu* 47 (To Consider the Long-term Depots as Foundations). These chapters clearly describe the principle of *zàng xiàng* 藏象/visceral manifestation. In the *Practical Dictionary of Chinese Medicine*, *zàng xiàng* 藏象/visceral manifestation is defined as "the manifestation of the activity of viscera and the bowels (and construction, defense, qi, blood,

---

1   Unschuld 2016 (*Ling shu*): 449

fluids, essence and spirit) in outwards signs; the Chinese medical physiology of the human body in which the viscera are understood to play a central role."[2] What is going on in the inside of the body and mind can be viewed on the outside, through observing changes in the pulse, complexion, abdominal tone, and along channel pathways. Through these external signs the physical can then work on what's going on in the inside. The Chinese didn't have x-rays, MRIs, EKGs or the range of modern medical technology, which forced physicians to develop very precise tools to observe changes in the external body, excretions, temperature changes, the shape of various structures such as ears, sternum, eyes, mouth and to listen to the voice and abdominal sounds. This led to a more "qualitative" type of diagnosis, one focused on movement rather than fixed measurements, reflecting Chinese philosophy and culture's central concerns about transformations (huà 化) and changes (biàn 變), and working with them to restore a smooth flow and harmonious function with the laws of the universe.

"A fractal is defined as a never-ending pattern. Fractals are infinitely complex patterns that are self-similar across different scales."[3] The smallest part has the same pattern and shape as the whole major picture. In Chinese medicine, there are several micro-systems that work in a fractal sense, reproducing the whole of the human body in miniature sub-systems that can be read in specific locations, such as at the cùn kǒu 寸口/inch-mouth location of the radial pulse. In addition, tongue diagnosis, abdominal diagnosis, the wǔ shū xué 五输穴/five transporting points can be said to be holographic or fractal. Later developments in Chinese medicine included micro-systems such as ear, scalp, head (based on ancient constellation maps), abdominal and hand acupuncture, where a specific region of the body reproduces the entire structure. This is the secret as to how the nine indicators (three positions

2   Wiseman and Ye 1998: 656
3   http://fractalfoundation.org/resources/what-are-fractals

and three depths) of the pulse can read a tripartite *sān jiāo* 三焦/triple burner map of the body/mind.

Chapter 47 (*Běn Zàng* 本臟/Foundation of Five Viscera) of the *Ling shu* is one of the essential chapters for understanding the principle of *zàng xiàng* 藏象/visceral manifestation. Visceral manifestation is one of the earliest systematic approaches focused on how the five yin viscera are viewed as being the foundation of human life and health. *Ling shu* 47, explains how the *wǔ zàng* 五臟/five yin viscera manifest in external symptoms, focusing on shape and size of body structures and sense organs, and symptoms such as breathing and thirst. Before modern screening technologies, Chinese physicians had to hone their observation skills to see signs of internal disharmonies and changes in the pulse, abdomen, complexion, skin qualities, sense organ/limb shape, dimensions, positions, and other qualities. This led to amazingly accurate diagnoses that allowed for effective medical practice. Sadly, few in our profession are even aware that this principle is a guiding light for practice, which is why we must make the argument for deep study of the classics. We find the following quote:

> Those whose five long-term depots (zàng/yin viscera) are all small, they rarely fall ill, but suffer from a "haggard heart", with much worry and agitation. Those whose zàng/yin viscera are all big, they approach all tasks in a relaxed mind and rarely fall prey to agitation. Those whose five zàng are all elevated, they love to take up great projects. Those whose five zàng are sunken down, they love to mingle with people. (*Ling shu* 47)[4]

The text also discusses core relationships between the visible tissues and internal organs. In the following section, the *fǔ* 腑/bowels are discussed:

---

4   Unschuld 2016 (*Ling shu*): 458

Huang Di: I wish to be informed of what the six *fǔ* 腑/bowels correspond to.

Qi Bo: The lung corresponds to the skin. When the skin is thick, the large intestine is thick. When the skin is thin, the large intestine is thin. When the skin is relaxed, and if the abdominal cavity is big, the large intestine is big and long. When the skin is tight, the large intestine is tight and short. When the skin is smooth, the large intestine is extended. When skin and flesh cannot be separated, the large intestine is knotted.

The heart corresponds to the vessels. When the skin is thick, the vessels are thick. When the vessels are thick, the small intestine is thick. When the skin is thin, the vessels are thin. When the vessels are thin, the small intestine is thin. When the skin is slack, the vessels are slack. When the vessels are slack, the small intestine is big and long. When skin is thin and vessels passable and small, the small intestine is small and short. When all yang channel vessels are curved and bent, the small intestine is knotted.

One inspects the external correspondences to know the condition of the internal viscera. Then one knows what their illnesses are. (*Ling shu* 47)[5]

The *Ling shu ji shaoshi* 灵枢经校释, a commentary on the *Ling shu* writes that "the physical appearance refers to the associations of the human body with the five phases. In ancient times, the people distinguished men on the basis of their qi qualities into five types based on the system of the five phases. Hence, persons associated as having a physical appearance associated with the phase wood than people whose appearance is associated with the phase earth. They fall ill at different times because of the regularities of mutual generation (*shēng* 生) and overcoming (*kè* 剋), as well as

5   Unschuld 2016 (*Ling shu*): 458–459

opposing the requirements of the five phases. This is called 'the emergence of disease because of one's physical appearance'."[6]

In the *Ling shu*, physicians used the image of nature and correlated that with the *xiàng* 象/image of the human body. We observe that the "clinical gaze" of the physician is educated by studying the medical philosophy in these texts, unique to Han dynasty thought and philosophy; an inviolable connection of humankind with nature, in terms of laws, phenomena, and a series of patterns and relationships that are an unbroken chain. The secret to successful practice of Chinese medicine is in studying and embodying these relationships, then applying this medical philosophy to diagnosis and treatment. All illness is a result of losing one's resonance with the natural laws of yin/yang, five phases, and seasonal qi, and cure is restoring resonance with these laws.

> As long as the normal functions of the *zàng* 臟/yin viscera can be maintained, there is peace (health). Where the normal functions are diminished, there is disease. (*Ling shu* 47)[7]

The role of the physician from this perspective is based on the strength and *zhèng* 正/correct status of the *wǔ zàng* 五臟/five yin viscera. They are to be guarded, protected, and treated according to the methods of supplementation and drainage described elsewhere in the *Su wen* and *Ling shu*. In addition, we can use (in herbal medicine) the eight methods mentioned in the *Shang han lun*: *hé* 和/harmonization, *bǔ* 補/supplementation, *wēn* 溫/warming, *xiè* 瀉/draining, *xiāo* 消/dispersing, *tù* 吐/ejection (vomiting), *hàn* 汗/sweating, and *qīng* 清/clearing.

In this chapter, we see that the correspondences between natural law and its processes are fully reflected in the human entity, and harmonizing with these laws is what ensures health and allows one to avoid illness. However, extreme weather

---

6   Unschuld 2016 (*Ling shu*): 445
7   Unschuld 2016 (*Ling shu*): 457

conditions do create illnesses of their own that can afflict people, but one can prepare for such conditions by adapting to these changes through behavior, diet, clothing, or seeking proper shelter.

> ShaoYu: When heaven generates wind, that is not directed at a specific individual within the population. It's movement is entirely neutral, upright, and straightforward. Those who act against [the wind], they will get it [as a disease]. Those who avoid it will be in no trouble. It would be wrong to assume that [the wind] seeks a certain person. It is humans who act against [the requirements of the wind and hence get the disease].[8]

Rather than being superstitious about natural forces, the *Ling shu* advances the importance of human responsibility in following the Tao, the laws of nature.

> ShaoYu: Among the trees there are yin and yang [types], (facing the sun is yang, not facing the sun is yin), firm and brittle ones. Those that are firm [his knife] cannot enter. Those that are brittle, their bark is loose. When he reaches intersections with knots, his saw and axe will break... Those that are firm [their wood] is hard. Those that are brittle are harmed easily. How much does this apply to the differences among the timbers! The bark may be thick or thin, juice plentiful or minimal...
>
> All these possible scenarios will result in damage. How much more does this apply to man![9]

---

8   Unschuld 2016 (*Ling shu*): 438
9   Unschuld 2016 (*Ling shu*): 438-439

How the *Nan jing* views channel manifestation in body shape, size, limbs, proportions, front, back, upper, middle and lower burners

The *Nan jing*, *Su wen* and *Ling shu*, delineate the length of the channels , size and shape of the five *zàng* 臟/yin viscera and six *fŭ* 腑/bowels, and relate the external sense organs, size, shape and spacing to the condition of the internal viscera.[10] For example, a patient with long limbs will also have lengthened channels. If a channel pulse such as the gallbladder channel is weak, thin, or does not fill its appropriate indicator (discussed in *Nan jing* 18), one will also notice timidity or indecisiveness, a pallid complexion, or poor digestion. An insufficiency of liver qi in its channel will manifest in smaller, sunken eyes, with poor vision, and an insufficient pulse in the left guan position. A repletion of liver qi will manifest in intense gaze, larger eyes that bulge out of their sockets, and a wiry, replete pulse in the left guan position on the pulse. In addition, abdominal diagnosis, largely developed historically by Japanese physicians, will resonate with the internal viscera as described in the *Nan jing* with its five yin viscera map (see Appendix V).

When one studies the three texts in depth, one can visualize and internalize a view of the body incorporating front, back, upper, middle and lower burners, and 12 primary channel divisions. This in turn is expressed in the size, shape and relative location of associated sense organs, such as the ears in relation to the kidneys, or eyes in relation to the liver. And in addition, in the length of the limbs, along with the relative repletion or vacuity of channel qi visible in the texture of the skin, heat or cold, associated complexion and colors (pale white, angry red, purple), the strength of the abdominal muscles, sinews, bones

---

10 *Su wen* 18 has a commentary by Wang Bing in which he writes the total length of a "normal person's" conduit vessels to circulate through the body is 162 feet; *Ling shu* 14 describes the length of the bones, 17 describes the length of vessels, 31 and 32 the size and length of the intestines and stomach; *Nan jing* 23 describes the length of the vessels and 42 describes the dimensions of the intestines and stomach

(density and thickness), flexibility and clarity of the *xuè mài* 血脉/blood vessels. All of these give us a clear picture of our patients and allow us to come up with a resonant diagnosis that leads from the external view, *zàng xiàng* 臟象/visceral manifestation, to the interior viscera and structures. This is in contrast to the more "formal" diagnosis associated with TCM, "*zàng fǔ*" diagnosis, which relies on a chain of causality. For example, depressed liver qi leads to weakened spleen qi and stomach pain, therefore use *xiāo yáo sǎn*/free wanderer powder to treat this.

CHAPTER IX

THE PERFECT STORM
An Approach to Time in Chinese Medicine

When the ancients treated patients, they became familiar with the cycles of yin and yang and of time, and with the exhalations of qi from mountain, forest, river and marsh. They discerned the patient's age, body weight, social status, style of life, disposition, likes, feelings, and vigor. In accordance with what was appropriate to these characteristics, and avoiding what was not, they chose among drugs, moxa, acupuncture, lancing with the stone needle, decoctions and extracts. They straightened out old habits and manipulated patterns of emotions. Feeling their way, missing no opportunity and constantly adapting, in their reasoning there was not a hair-breadth's gap. They would go on to regulate the patient's dress, rationalize his/her diet, change his/her living habits, and follow the transformation of his/her emotions, sometimes treating according to environmental factors, sometimes according to individual factors.

Shen Kuo, Good Prescriptions by Su and Shen
(Su Shen liangfang), 12th century[1]

---

1   Scheid 2007: 42–43

If one reads the *Nan jing* from beginning to end, one begins to see that the author of this work is focusing on the phenomenon of time and its influence on human health and disease. Based on *Su wen* 3, the *Nan jing* expands on the principle of restoring the natural, orderly progression of time in the body and mind, by observing and correcting patterns of function. According to Nathan Sivin, "It is the harmoniously alternating interplay of opposites that forms time; it is time that underlies cosmic process; and it is cosmic process that provides a pattern for human reflection and conduct."[2] Chinese medicine emphasizes patterns of function through time more than specific structures of organs and cells, and it is these patterns that form the basis for diagnosis and treatment.

Approaches to time in Chinese medicine

We live in a time where reforming health care is a central issue in the United States. A few of the most pressing problems are the insufficient time that medical professionals spend with their patients, and an overemphasis on pharmacological or surgical solutions to complex health issues. Chronic, long-term illnesses have become an increasing burden on health care professionals, requiring more in-depth approaches to care that demand increased time and attention. A small but growing group of health care professionals are organizing their practices to spend more time with patients, and offering tools such as education, lifestyle and dietary counseling, and alternative approaches to managing chronic illness.

Chinese medicine has a large role to play in this sector as well, as one of our chief strengths is the comprehensive approach to health care delineated by Shen Kuo in the opening quote of this chapter, nine centuries ago. Even in modern times, Chinese medical practitioners tend to spend a greater

---

2   Sivin 1987: 151

amount of time with patients and address many of the issues that contribute to their complaints.

Time is the secret of Chinese medicine. There is an editorial in the *New York Times* by Neil Shubin entitled "January is the Cruelest Month"[3] on the topic "seasonal affect disorder." The article discusses how our internal clocks respond to the position of the sun in the sky, length of the day, lunar cycles, and how we have our own inner cycles and rhythms. *Su wen* Chapter 3 states: "As for the yang qi, this is like heaven and the sun. If the sun were to lose its location, then this would reduce longevity, and his physical appearance would not be refined."[4]

Chinese physicians throughout the long history of Chinese medicine carefully observed all these complex cycles which occur, and are discussed in *Su wen* in Chapters 69–77 in great detail. Today we observe changes in herbal prescriptions and treatment recommendations when the stem and branch transformations of *wǔ yùn liù qì* 五運六氣/five movements six qi theory, would result in the local climate and weather moving through warming and cooling cycles.

> While heat waves and droughts are common complaints during the early to middle Jin, this period begins to shift towards increasingly harsh and freezing winters in the later Jin.
>
> 故水本寒 寒急則水冰如地而能載物 水發而雹雪 是水寒亢極反似克水之土化 是謂兼化也
>
> Therefore the root of water is cold, and if the cold is severe then the water freezes like the earth and is able to fill up things, and then the water comes forth as hail and snow. This water is cold in the extreme and contrarily surpasses and subdues the earthly changes of water, and this is called simultaneous change.

---

3   Shubin 2013
4   Unschuld and Tessenow 2011: 62

經所謂 金木水火土 運行之類 寒暑燥濕風火 臨御之化 則天
道可見 民氣可調

What the classics call metal, wood, water, fire, and earth, they
are the types of elemental-movements and phases. As for
cold, heat, dry, damp, wind, and fire, they are the changes of
lín yù 臨御 (imperial governance). Then if the heavenly dao
can appear the people's qi can be harmonized.[5]

There are various applications of this theory in other clinical
texts. The *Shang han lun* speaks about how certain illnesses
associated with the six channels resolve, recur, intensify, or
weaken at specific times of day. That is sequential diagnosis.
There is also the idea in the *Su wen* of bringing the human being
into harmony with the present heaven/earth conformation
(calendrical, seasonal, 24-hour, 12- and 60-year cycles).
That is why we have systems with horary points or balance
five-phase cycles, seasonal cycles, host qi (*zhǔ qì* 主氣) and
guest qi (*kè qì* 客氣). Host qi means the normal seasonal qi
where you live. For example, normal winter temperatures in
Boulder, Colorado, will be a high of 41 degrees and a low of 17
degrees and will have fluctuations from the 60s to below 0. In
some years, there will be unusually warm winters (and we are
seeing more and more warmth due to climate change) which
will affect one's health, and there will be abnormally cold years.
You also have the phenomenon that the autumn or summer
will last too long and winter will begin too late. Then the guest
qi "overrides" the host qi and you have a long autumn and a
short winter. It is also possible that the host qi is too strong
and gets cold much too early, say in October, and it may stay
cold all the way into May or June and will have variance on the
seasons, and this has catastrophic effects on human health.

Weather changes in southern California are far more subtle
than they are in Colorado. When there are weather changes in
wind direction, humidity, air pressure, and climatic air masses,

---

5   Welden 2015: 218

yin or yang, it will affect the human bio-organism, and the body will try to respond to that change. If it can't respond effectively it will cause digestive problems, joint pain, and contraction of wind or cold. In other words, humans respond like plants or animals. When a cold winter is coming, animals intuitively know to grow thicker coats. Ants know how to store food earlier in the autumn. How do they "know" this? Nature has a form of intelligence. Modern culture may define intelligence as something confined to the brain but it permeates the body and is expressed through what the Chinese called our *zàng* 臟 or visceral systems. The Chinese don't just attribute intelligence to the brain, but to the five yin visceral systems of liver, heart, lung, spleen and kidney. We see intelligence in plants on how they respond, follow and move with the sun and how they open and close when the sun is up and down. It's amazing stuff and has been under our noses all this time. The truth is that the Chinese have looked at this very carefully and it intimately informs medicine. That means we also need to involve ourselves in these natural phenomena to understand them, and in turn, it helps us understand Chinese medicine at a deeper level. We have to live with these phenomena. When students want to study the pulse, I tell them to go to the area of San Diego known as Torrey Pines. On the high bluffs overlooking the ocean you can watch sets of waves roll in. Depending on the wind, the swells and storms out at sea or calm weather will create different wave lengths, sets of waves, directions, choppiness and smoothness. Every surfer knows this as "a good set" or "a bad set." Pulse phenomena are similar to this. The pulse can be choppy, flat, flooding, fast, or slow, it is the same "breathing" of the earth through winds and of the sea, the flow of the tides, with the moon lunar cycles working inside us all the time. Its right under our noses and if we are not aware of it and we don't look at ourselves in this way, we aren't going to see it. When we work with time, we synchronize with time to restore our health. People don't understand why acupuncture works so well with fertility—it's because acupuncture is a great tool for restoring normal ovulation and menstrual cycles.

In Chinese medicine, different levels of time are discussed: cyclic time, cosmic time, sidereal time, solar and lunar time, seasonal time, and, most uniquely, human visceral time, based on the flow of qi, blood, defense and construction through specific cycles that are modulated by a complex system of internal clocks.

When discussing Chinese medicine and its role in modern life, it can be argued that one of its essential strengths is its comprehensive medical philosophy, and specifically its approach to time. The understanding of change and its transformations in time is a common thread in such classical texts as the Yi jing 易经 (Classic of Change), and is expressed in such areas of study as astronomy, agriculture, calligraphy, military strategy and self-cultivation practices. The view of the phenomena of nature as movement and pattern rather than a fixed viewing point is pervasive throughout Chinese history. It is the core of how the Chinese traditionally viewed medicine, before Western medicine and science became a major influence on Chinese culture.

When we study the classical medical texts, we find an emphasis on patterns and the cyclic nature of symptoms, leading to stasis, decay, inflammation, exhaustion of yang, depression, accumulation, distortion of channel flow. In the life cycle of most plants, there is the movement from the core seed stage to sprouting in springtime, to leaves and flowers in summer, to fruition in late summer and early autumn, and to decay or death in late autumn and winter, returning back to the original seed state. All living beings, whether plant or animal, follow similar patterns of growth, fruition, and decay. Chinese medicine is based on observation of these life cycles and their associated transformations. The human being is seen as a microcosm and reflection of the greater dynamics in nature. Each living being has a particular lifespan, heart and breathing rate, metabolism, digestion suitable for specific foods, and sleep-wake cycle that distinguishes it from every other species. In addition, each living organism interacts with the environment in specific ways, and must maintain both internal and external equilibrium in order to prosper, reproduce, and remain healthy. For all life forms other than humanity, this is an automatic process governed by instinct and natural law. Human beings, gifted with free will, paradoxically must choose to live with or against natural cycles. Chinese medicine first and foremost teaches a philosophy based on safeguarding and prolonging health called nourishing life (*yǎng shēng* 养生). The first three chapters of the *Su wen* are based on instructions for living in harmony with the seasons and harmonizing emotions to avoid damage to the body and mind. As the *Ling shu* states, the human being is envisioned as a microcosm of heaven and earth, and subject to the same laws:

> Heaven is round, the earth is rectangular. Man's head is round, his feet are rectangular. Heaven has sun and moon; man has two eyes. The earth has nine regions; man has nine orifices. Heaven has wind and rain; man has joy and rage. Heaven has thunder and lightning; man has the sound of his voice. Heaven has the four seasons; man has the four limbs. Heaven has five tones; man has the five long term depots... These are the correspondences between humanity and heaven and earth. (*Ling shu* chapter 71 *Xié Kè* 邪客/Evil Visitors)[6]

Human beings also are influenced by time within the society and culture in which they live. For example, a society may use a solar or lunar calendar, agricultural rhythms (sowing, cultivating, harvesting), animal herding (nomadic societies), industrial methods (clocks, transportation, assembly lines), or there is the informational, post-industrial society, with its rapid movement of digital information, contributing to excessive speed, stress, and anxiety. One can never catch up in this culture because digital rhythms move faster

---

6   Unschuld 2016 (*Ling shu*): 635

than biological time. The body clocks become confused and distorted, as in jet lag or night shifts at work, as we become more divorced from natural rhythms.

With our increased reliance on digital time, and the continued movement into the background of natural time determinants to human activity, people have difficulty keeping up with the artificial schedules (crossing time zones, working night shifts, undertaking late night studying for exams, postponing sleep, eating), leading to confusion and distortion in our body clocks, which is expressed through chaos in functional health, such as bowel rhythms, menstrual cycles, and sleep cycles. This in turn can lead to emotional and psychological disturbances, fatigue, disorientation, and an increased reliance on drugs that create their own distortion of circadian rhythms. As discussed in Chapter 3 of this book, when we use replacement therapies through drug analogues that mimic natural processes to stimulate "energy," bring on sleep or quiescence, or alter our moods, we risk becoming dependent on external substances that are now embodied in our visceral systems. In addition, time distortion is one of the main factors in the upsurge of autoimmune diseases and allergies.

The *Nan jing* and diagnosis

The *Nan jing*, in the Fiftieth Difficult Issue, speaks about the transference of internal evils according to the five-phase cycle via the channels between the viscera and bowels. Each viscera and bowel has a terrain of emotions, functions, physiology, and so on, that is healthy when operating harmoniously with other visceral systems, and unhealthy when overacting on other systems or weakened so that other systems dominate it. Nigel Wiseman's translation of "evil" for *xié* 邪 rather than "pathogen" acknowledges that in this view, it is the unhealthy relationship itself that is evil, not a pathogen per se. The violation of the space of a viscera, bowel, or channel means the body and mind have lost their dynamic equilibrium. Thus, the Nan jing describes five types of internal evils as follows: weak evils, thief evils, repletion evils, vacuous evils, and correct evils. Correct evils are defined as those that are contracted by a specific channel or viscera according to predictable evils, such as wind damaging the liver, or fire damaging the heart. The other evils have to do with the generating and controlling cycles of the five phases, and may develop due to emotional, seasonal, or other evils that are transferred according to phase, constitutional factors, or disharmonies of the viscera and bowels that become entrenched. When emotions or functions of the five yin viscera are disturbed by external or internal aberrations, illnesses may follow.

Chinese medicine has multiple models of pattern identification and differentiation, and flexibility is the key. Sometimes a Shang han lun, six-channel model may be best. Other times, a Nan jing five-phase model works best, as in the following case of a woman who suffered from a Parkinson's-like disease. She had severe tremors, seizures, sinew twitches, and difficulty speaking. It had progressed for several years, and possibly had been influenced by shock therapy treatments 30 or so years ago. When she tried to speak, she struggled to get the words out and would quickly become agitated. Her tongue was short, shriveled and red at the tip, with a yellow coating at the rear. Her body had shrunk over the years as well; she was very small with marked emaciation, and her right arm was frozen distally from the shoulder. Her fingernails and toenails were yellow, and her fingernails were ridged, while her fingers curled without coordination. At 65, her pulses were surprisingly strong, but according to Nan jing pulse analysis, the wood positions (liver and gallbladder positions) on the left wrist were relatively vacuous, while the inch (cùn) and foot (chǐ) positions were replete. The movement in the pulse wave indicated that the liver qi was counter-flowing upwards, invading the fire position (heart position at the cùn), and was then counter-flowing downwards, attempting to discharge through the kidneys. The liver was asked to do too much, so had lost its qi to the fire element (heart), and had to do the work of the kidney, which was drained of its qi and essence.

The philosophy of the *Nan jing* on these matters is that each of the five yin viscera has its position, qi, qualities, and function, and interacts with the other phases and viscera in a healthy or unhealthy way, via the generating (*shēng* 生) and control (*kè* 剋) cycles. When the qi of a phase overwhelms another due to imbalance (physiological or emotional)—or seasonal violation disrupts the normal order—this is considered to be a form of internally generated evil qi. Accordingly, in the description of the liver in the 41st difficult issue of the *Nan jing*, we see that the liver has "two lobes," or "two hearts:"

> Only the liver has two lobes. What does this correspond to? The liver is [associated with the] East and [with the phase of] wood. Wood [corresponds to] spring. [During this time of spring] all things come to life, they are still young and small. In their sentiments they are not [yet] close to anything. [The period of spring] moves away from the major yin [of winter] and it is still near to it. It is separate from the major yang [of summer], but is not far away from it. It appears to have two hearts. Hence, [the liver] has two lobes. This also corresponds to the leaves of the woods.[7]

As wood rests between water and fire, or spring between winter and summer, the liver functions and coordinates both the kidney and heart, which are connected by the *shǎo yīn* 少陰 channel. In this case, liver qi counterflows and attacks the heart (mother phase attacks child), and is undernourished by its mother phase, the kidney. Therefore, it is easily stressed (speech is associated with the heart), and its qi cannot rest in its proper place, so it bifurcates and alternates between the water and heart phases.

---

7   Unschuld 2016 (*Nan jing*): 345

For the above case, I suggested to the husband, who is also an acupuncturist, that he must strengthen the kidney, return the liver qi to its source (using the source point of liver channel), and return wood qi from the heart back to the liver (using the fire point on liver channel, Liver 2 (*xíng jiān* 行間), or wood point on fire channel, Heart 7 (*shén mén* 神門). In addition, a herbal prescription and lifestyle changes must be made to ground the liver in its source, using emotions, seasonal qi, foods, and meditation. This is one example of how we can apply five-phase theory from the *Nan jing* to the practice of Chinese medicine.

The Eighth Difficult Issue states, "All the channels are connected with the source qi (*yuán qì* 原氣)." This source qi fills all of the channels and circulates through the body, communicating essence (*jīng* 精) from one region to another. The channel system coordinates, supplies and drains the viscera and the bowels, maintaining a harmonious balance. When there is a loss of communication between the viscera and bowels, due to the channels being blocked, depleted, or shunted in a different direction, this may lead to what we describe as "illnesses of compensation." In other words, the necessary checks and balancing mechanisms are distorted, leading to over-activity in some viscera, and chaotic flow in the channels. Since the body must always maintain systemic balance, the patient develops a chronic disease of many facets, and because underlying it is a deep-set pattern, it is difficult to resolve without a treatment plan that addresses the underlying complex pathomechanisms. These undesirable patterns can then be addressed through herbal medicine, acumoxa, therapeutic exercises, and diet, along with regulation of daily activities, rest, and emotions.

Just as we humans develop emotional and psychological coping strategies, we may also develop these strategies at a physiological level as well. Many of these coping strategies may work temporarily, but end up being damaging to both emotional and physiological health in the long run. The body often serves as a conduit for the emotions in such symptoms as skin rashes, hemorrhoids, recurrent urinary tract infections, irritable bowel syndrome, and abdominal pain. Thoughts and emotions are sometimes mirrored in physiological processes (and vice versa) in an auto-feedback loop. Fixations and false strategies become embedded in the body, seen in abnormal posture, contracted muscles, arthritis, abnormal bowel rhythms, or marked weight gain. Just as people develop strategies to deal with emotional overload, they also self-medicate, using coffee, alcohol, recreational drugs, sex, hyper-exercise, overeating, and special diets to try to find balance or relief, but it is often done in an unconscious or unproductive fashion. It is the job of the Chinese medical physician to replace false strategies with healthy ones, to rectify past issues with the present, and to help project healthy new directions for the future.

The core of visceral manifestation theory is that diagnosis is based on what the body shows. The Chinese medical physician looks for patterns in handwriting, mode of dress and hairstyle, movement (walking, sitting, loud or soft movements), speech, perfume, and makeup. What is the patient projecting about themselves? Is it a true picture of what is inside, or a projection of an ideal? How does the patient approach their treatment? Do they take responsibility for their own health? How many doctor visits have they had? How many procedures? How much medication do they take? When evaluating our patients, we can keep in mind the words of Huang Di in chapter 39 of the *Su wen*:

> When one is angry, then the qi rises. When one is joyous, then the qi relaxes. When one is sad, then the qi dissipates. When one is in fear, then the qi moves down... When one is frightened, then the qi is in disorder. When one is exhausted, then the qi is wasted. When one is pensive, then the qi lumps together.[8]

---

8   Unschuld and Tessenow 2011: 594

When I treat complex cases, I often draw a "flow chart" for my patients, showing how the condition developed over time, often beginning with an initial, often overlooked, trauma; for example, a woman in her forties whose health never recovered after a bout of mononucleosis in college, suffering from irregular menstrual cycles, severe fatigue, bloating after eating, poor digestion, and disturbed sleep. A number of factors combine from climate, season, emotional stress, constitutional weakness, diet, and unresolved symptoms to create "the perfect storm" that manifests as a disease. This can be drawn as a timeline extending as a string of symptoms and disease factors from the past, to the present pattern using a system of diagnosis—whether five-phase theory, viscera-bowel, six-channel or another type of pattern differentiation—that can be used as a relational model. This model allows both the physician and the patient to intervene in the body-mind system providing new stimuli to open communication in the channels and restore homeostasis. In the *Nan jing*, acupuncture treatment is designed to restore disturbed order to the channel and visceral systems through sophisticated five-phase treatment strategies.

The value of the above methodology recorded in the *Nan jing* is that it allows the physician to view a patient's health and disease patterns as a process, a movement in time, rather than just a snapshot taken at one point in time, and then trying to base a diagnosis and treatment plan on it. The physician, by observing the past, is able to project the future course of health and illness.

Chronobiology in the *Su wen* and the *Nan jing*

The Chinese applied cyclic ideas of time (to the microcosm of) the life-maintaining order of the human body, in phase with the environment and with the individual's emotional and rational processes. This seemed to constitute a remarkably articulated nest of cycles, with the life trajectory of the mayfly or the diurnal rhythm of the human body representing the smallest wheel, and, as the largest, the practically infinite great cycle—from the beginning until the end of time— integrating all the astronomical periods, all the small cycles turning within it like a superbly complicated train of gears.[9]

The next aspect to investigate is the periodicity of symptoms. In five movements and six qi theory (wǔ yùn liù qì 五運六氣), the Chinese recognized that all sentient beings and phenomena had internal clocks that measured cycles of change, birth, growth, decay, and death. Symptom patterns were recognized as being dependent on the variables of the 24-hour clock of the internal viscera, seasons, year, and other cycles. Symptoms such as heart palpitations were observed to see when they occurred to associate them with the rise and fall of qi in specific channels and in the bowels and viscera. Medicines and acupuncture points were chosen to coordinate with the best times in regard to the rise and fall of qi in treatment. The pulse was also seen to vary at different times of day, season or other natural cycles. As the sun rose from dawn to its zenith in the sky, the yang qi would increase and strengthen in the pulse. As it sank in the sky towards dusk, yang qi would decrease and the yin quiescent qi of nighttime would increase.

Circadian rhythms are extremely influential. Just watch them change and morph into new patterns, constantly flowing, changing like the sea. Neurotransmitters and hormones, moods, ideas, and emotions rise and fall. One day you feel cloudy-minded and distracted, the next evening, you are inspired to compose sonnets. A dream brings you a new direction and realization. The next day, your body aches, you are tired, and cannot concentrate. On the following day, the air is dry, the sunlight strong and you awaken early with vibrant energy. However, you are also more impatient, and find it hard to make decisions or concentrate on one issue at a time.

---

9   Sivin 1987: 152

One day you want to stay put, the next day you want to dance. Appetites change, even perceptions of color change. Plants change, the growth patterns of flowers change, even in a vase. Yin and yang flow and interact, the visceral systems exchange, harmonize and clash, and symptoms appear and disappear.

While it may seem to be common sense to live with the dynamic flow of time, which is clearly outlined in the *Su wen* and other Chinese medical texts, most human beings want to "do what they want" and in this way affirm their individual existence. Interestingly, we often act against our own health by pushing too hard, enjoying foods that reinforce ill health, so that we need to be educated in how to re-synchronize ourselves with natural rhythms. In the *Su wen*, this is defined as "going with the flow" (*shùn* 順) as opposed to "against the flow" (*nì* 逆). Going against the flow is seen as the root of all disease.

> But some clocks have not changed with technology, human interchange or commerce. Virtually every part of us—all our organs, tissues and cells—are set to a rhythm of day and night. Kidneys slow down at night. That's a wonderful trait if you want to minimize trips outside of bed. The human liver works slowest in the morning hours, meaning the cheapest dates would be at breakfast.
>
> How do these biological rhythms come about? We carry more than two trillion clocks inside of us. Our genetic clocks are set to the sun by our brains and our eyes. Light entering our eyes triggers a signal that ends in a tiny patch of cells in the brain. This brain region then emits hormones that coordinate the clocks in the different cells of the body. Mess with this system and things go awry really fast.[10]

The great scholar-physicians of China tracked these changes and recorded them in the classical texts, meditations on human life and health. Ancient texts such as the *Nan jing* are

---

10 Shubin 2013

meditations on the relationship of human life to the visible universe, using the rubric of time to connect everything together. There is a different world of time in the texts from the periods of the Warring States and Han dynasty, and we must live this chronotope in order to be effective physicians. We must learn to look beyond a model that promises instant relief or an instant cure; health and disease ebb, flow, process, and follow cycles. This is the crux of how to properly apply Chinese medicine today.

CHAPTER X

GǍN YÌNG 感應/RESONANCE:
An Essential Principle of Classical Chinese Medicine

黃帝問於歧伯曰： 經脈十二者，外合於十二經水，
而內屬於五藏六府。

Huang Di asked Qi Bo:

*The twelve conduit/stream vessels link up with the twelve
stream waters outside, and they are connected with the
five long-term depots and six short-term repositories
inside.*

(*Ling shu* 12)[1]

The theory of resonance can be thought of as a cognitive map
for understanding the universe in terms of ancient Chinese
philosophy. The interconnectedness of *yuán wù* 原物/
multiple phenomena in specific ways, through application of
heaven/human/earth triad and yin/yang theory, has been a
cornerstone of Chinese medicine since its early origins.

One specific example of resonance appears in *Ling shu*
12 (*Jīng Shuǐ* 經水/The Conduit/Stream Waters) where the
mapping of the *jīng mài* 經脈/conduit/stream vessels in a
human being is compared to the rivers, their basins, and
the overall mapping of China. In turn, this resonates with the

---

1   Unschuld 2016 (*Ling shu*): 215

human being, who is seen as a landscape with mountains, rivers, lakes, valleys, and natural landmarks. According to Paul Unschuld, the term *jīng* 經 originally described the weft of woven tissue, and he described such "weaving" as economy and culture.[2] *Jīng* 經 also describes the major rivers and streams that supply water and irrigation and crops, as well as the transportation of goods on boats and barges. So in the human being, *jīng* 經 are seen as channels ("stream vessels") that allow transportation of vital substances through the body and support the various structures and functions so vital to human life. *Jīng* 經 are also seen as a system of informational transfer, according to Sandra Hill in her book *Chinese Medicine from the Classics*.[3] They provide the structure and form of the human body and its conscious expression as the *wǔ zhì* 五志/ five minds (*hún* 魂, *yì* 意, *pò* 魄, *zhì* 志 and *shén* 神).

> Now, the stream waters receive water and transmit it. The five long-term depots unite the spirit qi with the *hún* 魂 and *pò* 魄 souls and store them. The six short-term repositories (bowels) receive grain and transmit it; they receive the qi and disperse them. The *jīng mài* 經脈/conduit/stream vessels receive the blood and circulate it. (*Ling Shu* 12)[4]

Another example of resonance is in the work of Li Dong-yuan (1180–1251 CE). His theory of banking up the spleen and stomach was based on a way of thinking he no doubt developed under the influence of environmental and political influences from his home on the central plains of China. This area had been abandoned by the Mongol conquerors in the mid-13th century. The central plains and river basins of China were centers of agriculture and commerce, associated with the center (*zhōng* 中) of China, and in turn with the earth phase of five phase theory, and the *zhōng jiāo* 中焦/central burner of the spleen and stomach. The *dì* 地/earth/soil resonated with

---

2   Unschuld 2016 (*Ling shu*): 215
3   Hill 2014: 167
4   Unschuld 2016 (*Ling shu*): 216

the central burner's role of fermenting foodstuffs into qi and blood. The central *pí* 脾/spleen viscus separated *qīng qì* 清氣/clear qi and *zhuó qì* 濁氣/turbid qi and was also the location where the essential post-natal qi was created.

Yìng 應/resonance informs both acupuncture/moxibustion therapy and internal/"herbal" medicine. Through acupuncture and moxibustion, we send signals to the body/mind to restore a state of dynamic homeostasis and attempt to redirect the flow of qi and blood in the channels and network vessels to obtain this state. Once this "memory" of homeostasis is re-awakened, the body/mind will attempt to re-adjust to return to a balanced state and spontaneously heal itself. In herbal medicine, we similarly create combinations of plants, animal parts and minerals to reconstruct a virtual state of health by superimposing the combination of medicinals that will restore this homeostasis.

In the 21st century, this work has become more challenging because of the extreme degrees of disconnection of human beings from the natural world. According to Moises Velasquez-Manoff, in his book *Epidemic of Absence* (2013), the human body and mind are not designed to adapt to these artificial ways of life, including diet (chemicalized, bioengineered, devitalized foods), work and study schedules (jet lag, disturbed sleep cycles, excessive work at nighttime and late night study), unregulated lifestyles, centralized heating and cooling in buildings, synthetic building materials and clothing, fast transportation, and the rapidly increasing speed of digital information transferral. For many people, Chinese medicine and other traditional systems are difficult to understand because they are based on a pre-industrial era focused on natural science, on observing natural cycles, habitats, animal, plant and mineral kingdoms, flows of water in streams and rivers, ocean tides, and lunar, solar, and planetary cycles. The practice of Chinese medicine as a way of life (*yǎng shēng* 養生) requires a re-immersion in an observance and participation in these natural cycles.

> Heaven has the qi of the four seasons. The earth has the
> requirements of the five directions. The people differ in where
> the live, how they dress, and what they eat. In treatment one
> distinguishes between needling, cauterization, and drugs.
> Hence the sages either orientated themselves on the qi of
> heaven, or they acted in accordance with the requirements
> of the cardinal direction, or they followed the disease of
> the respective person. Hence they sometimes used needles,
> cauterization, or toxic drugs, in other cases [they treated
> with] exercises or massage. (Zhang Zhi-cong's commentary
> on *Su wen* 12)[5]

The ancient Chinese observed that the different regions of
China produced different therapies, which are explained
in chapter 12 of the *Su wen* (*Yì fǎ fāng yí lùn* 異法方宜論/
Discourse on Different [Therapeutic] Patterns Suitable [for
Use in Different] Cardinal Points). It begins with Huang Di
asking Qi Bo, "When physicians treat diseases, one identical
disease may be treated differently in each case, and is always
healed. How is that?" Qi Bo responds, "Physical features of
the earth let it be this way."[6] Qi Bo goes on to explain that
massage, body work and dietetics in the central earth region,
moxibustion (*jiǔ ruò* 灸焫, meaning to cauterize) in the north,
therapy with pointed stones (bloodletting) in the eastern coastal
regions, herbal medicine in the west and the nine needles (*jiǔ
zhēn* 九針) of acupuncture south all developed in regions of
China where they served as "antidotes" for the predominating
conditions of their associated region. Each environment was
associated with the four directions and the central plains,
each with their specific characteristics that nurtured different
bodily constitutions, but also promoted tendencies to specific
types of disease.

Similar principles were at work in Greco-Arabic medicine. In Hippocrates' *Airs, Waters and Places,* he describes

---

5   Unschuld and Tessenow 2011: 217
6   Unschuld and Tessenow 2011: 211

environments in terms of soil quality, prevailing wind directions, exposures to bodies of water, hours of sunlight, and protection by mountain peaks. These environments in turn supported health and nurtured illness in specific proportions, which then led to specific therapies to counter these illnesses. China, and Tibet (along with Qinghai and Yunnan provinces) are known as "the land of herbs." From what I've observed, studying and practicing herbal wildcrafting in the Rocky Mountains of Colorado and New Mexico and the deserts and mountains of California, is that the more extreme environments produce a higher potency of medicinal substances in the plant kingdom. In high altitude regions, one will notice a yin/yang polarity from one side of a canyon or mountain ridge to another. On the sunny or southern-facing side, there is much more sun exposure, and the soil is drier, and the plants are desert-like, with a warm, desiccating nature. On the northern, shady side, the soil is moist, especially where streams are flowing, there are trees and better water retention, so the plants have a more yin, moistening nature (there are exceptions, such as zé xiè 泽泻/plantago root, which grows in wet, swampy areas, but expels excess moisture from the lower burner). The extremes of sunlight and shade (where temperatures may vary several degrees during the day), daytime and nighttime (where temperatures will rise and fall up to 50 degrees in a single day), summer and winter, produce hardy plants with profound medicinal properties.

We can view classical Chinese medicine as a body of knowledge with resonant properties. While different theories were often espoused in the *Su wen*, a heterogeneous text with several authors, the end result was a *jīng* 經/web of theories that are interrelated, a "hypertext" approach with commentaries that resembles modern point-and-click links on the internet. It can also be compared with the *Talmud*, a text with multiple commentaries written over several centuries, each seeming to be in dialogue with each other. Texts such as the *Su wen*, *Nan jing* and *Shang han lun* have been re-interpreted through commentaries by great physicians throughout the long history of the field.

Clinically, *gǎn yìng* 感應/resonance is expressed, after a complete examination of pulse and other palpation diagnoses, questioning, observing tongue and complexion, in the choice of treatment to correct the flow of qi and blood and restore the natural order of the channel system. Our tools are needles, moxa, or herbal medicine, along with bringing the lifestyle of the patient back in synchronicity with their circadian rhythms and heaven/earth cycles. When a person is resonant and harmonious with their own self, it becomes easier to "go with the flow'" with the changes that occur in seasonal qi, day and night, lunar cycles of 28 days, and the qualities of specific years. This vital concept of *wǔ yùn liù qì* 五運六氣/five periods and six qi is discussed in chapters 69–77 of the *Su wen*. With this understanding, we can then predict where abnormal weather patterns can disrupt human health and lead to disease.

CHAPTER XI

CASE HISTORIES

Throughout my long career, I always have tried to get the most information about my patient, then filter a diagnosis into one that was simple without being simplistic (Einstein: make your theory as simple as possible, but no simpler), one that found the core in the midst of complexity. In *Su wen* 76, this is called the *yuán wù bǐ lèi* 援物比類 principle, which is to draw on the facts and compare the likes—or as Yu Chang (1585–1664) and Cheng Goupeng (1662–1735) taught as "awakening the mind" (*xīn wú* 心唔), which is "a moment when after much study and application, even the most difficult becomes simple and clear."[1] As a practitioner of both acupuncture/moxibustion and herbal medicine, two interrelated but distinct disciplines, I've had to investigate appropriate diagnostic paradigms for each. For acupuncture, I've relied on channel theory from the acupuncture classics, especially the *Nan jing*, and for herbal medicine, the *liù jīng biàn zhèng* 六經辨證/six-channel pattern differentiation (theory) in the *Shang han lun*. I read the pulse as my primary diagnostic method, but also look at the tongue, palpate the abdomen, observe the complexion, listen to the voice, detect body and breath scents, and (following the *Ling shu*) look at the shape of the sense organs on the face, shape of the trunk, length of limbs, fingers and toes, look for discolorations, skin eruptions and visible blood vessels along the channels. Then, and only then, do I ask the patient to

---

1   Scheid 2009: 122

tell me what is bothering them. This way I avoid the bias of being influenced by a biomedical diagnosis or the results of blood tests, CT scans, and other mainstream medical testing. I also encourage patients to reframe their symptoms as a moving picture, contextualizing their symptoms in a greater holistic view. I feel it is very important to stimulate a person's self-awareness, both through the diagnostic process, and through treatment itself.

Case history 1

May 25, 2017 Patient is 37 years old, has four children, three under five, the youngest being 19 months. Nineteen days ago, her mouth suddenly was drooping on the left side, her tongue felt numb, as well as the left side of her face. She was diagnosed by a Western physician with Bell's Palsy, put on prednisone for five days and an antiviral drug for seven days. Three days before the Bell's Palsy attack, she was given a depo-provera shot to avoid getting pregnant yet again, since she had four small children and didn't feel she could handle another child. The patient had not had a period since August 2015. She sustained a small skull fracture after hitting the back of her head a few years ago, and lost her sense of taste after that. Now she was tearing up uncontrollably, and finding it difficult to eat or drink because of her drooping mouth and face muscles. She was experiencing occasional headaches, and echoing in her ear on the left side. She had lost 20 pounds in the last few months.

Her tongue had a very dark red tip, the tongue body had a white coating and a washed-out purple color. The pulse was large and hollow in all positions, with sogginess. The abdomen was soft and pliable.

In Chinese medicine, Bell's Palsy is connected with an external attack of wind evil, often contracted by patients suffering from internal *láo sǔn* 勞損/vacuity taxation. In this case, the patient was depleted by having several children in succession, and it was notable that she had not had a period in two years. The depo-provera shot is known to have many powerful side-effects, including numbness and weakness on one side of the body, severe headaches, fever, puffy swelling of the extremities, and disruption of the menstrual cycle in terms of heaviness, pain, and loss of regularity. The pulse indicated an exterior attack of wind, but the formlessness and hollowness of the pulse indicated internal vacuity and susceptibility to wind, and a more dramatic reaction to the depo-provera. This was a *tài yáng* disorder, where wind evil had penetrated the channels of the face. Underneath, there was qi and blood vacuity with cold blood stasis accumulating in the lower burner.

My treatment was to needle alternate sides, LI 4 (*hé gǔ*), K 6 (*zhào hǎi*), Lu 7 (*liè quē*), TB 5 (*wài guān*) and GB 41 (*zú lín qì*). I also needled stomach channel points on the face, and used a moxa pole on the affected areas. In addition, I needled and applied moxa to the abdomen, putting moxa on the needles at Ren 6 (*qì hǎi*) and St 30 (*qì chōng*). Her herb formula was unmodified *gé gēn tāng*/kudzu decoction. I also gave her a moxa pole to apply to facial areas at home.

We had a follow up visit on June 2, 2017. There was much visible improvement with the eyes, no tearing up, the mouth and face were not drooping, the headache and ear "echos" were gone. The tongue body was swollen, the tip was less red, and there was a thick coating. She had had difficulty eating her normal diet since the depo-provera shot, and this may have impacted her spleen and stomach. The pulse, however, was now rapid and wiry, especially the right guan pulse. The left-hand pulse was rapid, short contracted and wiry as well. I kept her on the same herb formula for a few more days, and then we switched to *chái hú guì zhī tāng*/bupleurum and cinnamon twig decoction. For acupuncture, I needled (alternate sides) the *chōng* and *dài mài* "master-couples," Sp 4 (*gōng sūn*) and P 6 (*nèi guān*), SI 3 (*hòu xī*) and Bl 62 (*shēn mài*), with H 7 (*shén mén*). We also repeated the facial and abdominal points, with moxa.

At the next appointment on June 12, 2017, the facial symptoms had improved. The tongue still had a thick coating, but the tip was less red. The pulse had switched to being contracted, small, beady and tight. I needled alternate sides TB 5 (*wài guān*) and GB 41(*zú lín qì*), K 6 (*zhào hǎi*)/Lu 7 (*liè quē*) and LI 4 (*hé gǔ*), with H 7 (*shén mén*) again, along with a few face points, and the abdominal points as before. I switched the herbal formula to *guì zhī fú líng wán*/cinnamon twig and poria pill, to deal with the internal static blood.

At this point, we found out that the patient may have been pregnant at the time of the depo-provera shot, which raised both of our concerns that this could be a dangerous situation for the fetus, if indeed she was truly pregnant. Also, the shift on the pulse from floating and hollow to deeper, contracted and wiry/rapid was of great concern to me in this respect. On July 3, 2017, the patient had a miscarriage, with an empty sac, and heavy bleeding. She was mildly depressed, but her Bell's Palsy symptoms were completely alleviated. After this breakthrough bleeding, the pulse was overall deep, thin and rough, with some blockage on guan/chi on the left side. The tongue still had a very thick turbid coating. I needled alternate sides Sp 4 (*gōng sūn*)/P 6 (*nèi guān*), along with LI 10 (*shǒu sān lǐ*)/St 37(*shàng jù xū*) to regulate *yáng míng* and help clear the discharge of fetus and blood, with moxa and needles on the abdomen. I had the patient continue with *guì zhī fú líng wán*/cinnamon twig and poria pill.

At this point, the patient was satisfied with her progress. I recommended additional treatment to stabilize her *chōng* and *rèn* channels, and strengthen her spleen qi, and am hopeful she will return at some point in the near future to do so.

Case history 2

October 13, 2016 Patient is a young woman, 23 years old, diagnosed with Stills disease, an autoimmune disorder affecting the joints, rare but most common in young adults.

She had this diagnosis for eight months before coming in. It started with fevers twice a day, spiking to 104 degrees, frequent sore throat, with all joints and articulations painful. What was unique about the fever was that it could spike to 104 degrees, but then drop to 95 degrees after an attack (indicating exhaustion of kidney yang qi and essence). Sometimes after a fever at night, she would wake up in the morning freezing, then she'd have spontaneous sweating. Her white blood cell counts could rise up to 52,000, indicating an exaggerated immune response. In the past, her periods were very heavy, and always irregular, with cramping. She also was using an intrauterine device (IUD). She had been taking prednisone, 20 mg. at the time of the first treatment, but she had been as high as 60 mg., along with relatively high doses of methotrexate. She weighed 108 pounds, 18 pounds below normal, and was unable to gain weight. She was prone to frequent respiratory infections, coughing up yellow phlegm, and repetitive, angry skin rashes, exacerbated by the use of methotrexate. Before becoming ill, she had taken a trip to Costa Rica, where she was attacked by mosquitos. The tongue body was bright red with spots, especially at the tip and sides. Also, seven years ago, her brother died suddenly in an accident, and she was severely traumatized. The pulse was very soggy, forceless at the root, right chi pulse empty on the right. The left pulse was stronger, more forceful, and again weaker on depth.

My diagnosis was a combination *shào yīn/jué yīn* disorder, with *yáng míng* channel heat, damage to essence and yin fluids, and ministerial fire flaring out of control. Autoimmune disorders are shockingly common in young women in their early twenties. My long-term clinical experience with autoimmune disorders is that they tend to follow the seven-year cycles described in *Su wen* chapter 1, their origins often in disturbed menstrual cycles from their onset (at 12–14 years old). Many of these young women have had deep emotional traumas and over-treatment with antibiotics, hormones or vaccines when young, and they tend to shift into an exhausted state when they leave home for college, where they have no discipline with diet, sleep schedules, sexual activity, recreational drugs, partying or all-night studying for exams.

I have treated this young woman for eight months, and in that time, I've focused on treating the *jué yīn* and *shào yīn* channels, using point combinations such as alternate Liv 3 (*tài chōng*) with P 7 (*dà líng*), K 3 (*tài xī*) with H 7 (*shén mén*). I've also used liver/gallbladder divergent points such as Liv 8 (*qū quán*), GB 34 (*yáng líng quán*) and GB 1 (*tóng zǐ liáo*). I regularly have used back shu points, including kidney divergence such as Bl 11 (*dà zhù*), Bl 23 (*shèn shū*) (with moxa), and K 10 (*yīn gǔ*). To clear *yáng míng* heat, I have used points such as LI 11 (*qū chí*). We have had excellent results in reducing joint pain, increasing energy, reducing skin rashes, and reducing recurrence of colds and flu. However, this is an ongoing case in progress, which may take years of work. She is slowly weaning off the strong medications, so my use of herbal medicine has been relatively conservative. I started her with *wū méi wán*/mume pill, but for the last few months have used the combination of *shèn qì wán*/kidney qi pill 50 percent with *guì zhī fú líng wán*/cinnamon twig and poria pill 50 percent in honey pill form. Occasionally, when the fire was extreme, and sleep very disturbed with very rapid pulse, I've use *tiān wáng bǔ xīn dān*/emperor of heaven's special pill to tonify the heart to great effect.

Case history 3

Patient is a 35-year-old man. In 2009, he suffered from severe respiratory problems, with a lot of heat in the chest, sneezing, a sore throat and constant thirst. He easily became ill with colds and influenza, always with yellow to orange mucus. Digestion was sluggish, and he had gained weight to 275 pounds. He suffered from anxiety when he travelled for his work, had stiffness and soreness in his neck and shoulders. He sweated spontaneously, had heavy, forced breathing, and was unable to expectorate. He also suffered from hemorrhoids, occasional headaches, and neck pain. When sick, his cheeks would become flushed. He had also been diagnosed with fatty liver syndrome, tachycardia, and common ear infections with itching and hearing loss. Over the years, his weight had fallen, then gone up again dramatically. His lung symptoms had overall improved, but his blood circulation was poor, thinking unclear, and he had an occasional rapid heartbeat.

My diagnosis was triple yang disorder, *tài yáng/yáng míng/shào yáng*, with progressive damage to the yin layers of the body. Evil heat had damaged his lung and stomach yin, and greatly debilitated his spleen *tài yīn qi* transformation. My original treatment was to combine *tài yīn*, *shào yīn*, and *shào yáng* acupuncture points, including alternating Sp 9 (*yīn líng qúan*), K 7 (*fù liū*), Lu 5 (*yáng xī*) and Lu 6 (*piān lì*) (xi-cleft point), abdominal points with moxa below navel, St 40 (*fēng lóng*), Lu 2 (*yún mén*), St 2 (*sì bái*). His tongue was quite remarkable. The body was very red, and peeled in the front half. There was, on the unpeeled part, a thick, yellow and grey turbid coating, showing old turbid phlegm in the lungs and stomach. His root formula at the beginning was *bǎi hé gù jīn tāng*/lily bulb metal-securing decoction, which worked wonders and reduced his lung issues immensely. When there were pronounced phlegm symptoms, I'd use formulas such as *xiáo chái hú tāng*/minor bupleurum decoction combined with *wēn dǎn tāng*/warm gallbladder decoction, which was also very effective. This man has come in several times, on and off, over the years for different issues, and presently he is back in treatment primarily for anxiety, constipation, stiff neck and shoulders, migraines, sensitivity to heat, and sleep disturbance. His present formula (for triple yang disease) is *chái hú jiā lóng gǔ mǔ lì tāng*/bupleurum decoction plus dragon bone and oyster shell. A typical acupuncture point combination used is alternating K 2 (*rán gǔ*) with H 3 (*shào hǎi*), Liv 2 (*xíng jiān*) with P 3 (*qū zé*), TB 4 (*yáng chí*) with GB 40 (*qiū xū*), along with abdominal points.

Afterword

Ken Rose

I have long argued that Chinese medicine is first and foremost a cultural phenomenon. What this means is that it emerges from and depends on a dense matrix of cultural artifacts such as language and literature, philosophy and religion, food and farming—to name but a few of the more obvious ones. Thus, Chinese medicine has grown over many centuries from cultural roots that wind down through the soil of one of the earth's most durable civilizations. And how did the Chinese achieve this durability? Their medical traditions have played an important role in sustaining the well-being of both Chinese culture and the individuals who have thrived within it and caused it to thrive. It is indeed a robust and vital culture that today sustains a substantial proportion of the world's population, and a growing number of people today have come to depend on Chinese medicine for its health maintenance as well as for the management of disease.

Why? There are, no doubt, many answers, but at the root of the matter is one simple fact: it works. People turn more and more to acupuncture, herbal medicine, and the other modalities of Chinese medicine for relief from the pain and suffering of injury and illness; and more and more they find it works, even in cases when modern medicine has provided little help. Why is that? Chinese medicine provides practitioners and patients with a different way of thinking about health and disease, and this different way of thought leads to different and highly effective action when it comes to medical intervention.

Such consideration leads us to examine the traditions of knowledge and transmission of knowledge that have sustained Chinese medicine over the centuries. Among the most prominent of these traditions is that of the scholar-physician. To understand and appreciate the importance of the book you now hold in your hands (or read on your screen) you should see it in the context and framework of the scholar-physician. So what does this frame consist of? How can modern readers who may lack familiarity with the cultural context of ancient China come to terms with the requirement of understanding its implications?

There is far too much to say in answer to such questions, but for the purpose of providing an overview of this important framework, we can say that in the system of knowledge creation and transmission in which Chinese medicine has developed and moved through the past centuries, the scholar-physician has served as a critical node, both of knowledge creation and education. Scholar-physicians have collected, edited, revised, and reissued classical texts that have served as the vessels of knowledge transmission across generations. Many such texts have come to be identified with the names of doctors who not only stewarded the ancient texts but subjected the theories and methods they contain to ongoing trial and scrutiny in their own practices.

Thus, a highly practical approach emerged that blends theory and practice and recorded it, along with clinical results. And in this way, centuries of medical experience have been maintained and made available to generation after generation of students and practitioners. You may well be familiar with some of the names that live on in such literary traditions: Jiang Jie Bin; Li Shi Zhen; Zhang Ji; Sun Si-miao…to name but a few of the multitude of physicians who have toiled at such labor throughout Chinese history.

This work has really just begun in modern times and tongues. It is being conducted in the clinics and libraries of those who have come to recognize the essential importance of this approach. Among these clear-sighted individuals, one of the senior pioneers has been Z'ev Rosenberg. And in these pages that you have just read is nothing less than the contemporary expression of the ancient tradition of the physician-scholar engaged in the ongoing struggle of comprehending the challenges facing those who seek well-being and who follow ancient Chinese wisdom to obtain it.

Drugs and Their Effects on the Pulse

These are my observations from my clinical experience over a 35-year period.

Steroids (such as prednisone)

Steroids such as prednisone at first tend to influence the pulses to be flooding, rapid and slippery but without root. It is similar to taking a large dose of *fù zǐ* 附子/aconite root without other medicinals to temper it, and it consumes the yang qi and the *jīng* 精, the essence of the kidneys. Over time in terms of consuming *jīng* 精, it will thin the bones (associated with kidneys), cause premature aging, and interfere with separation of clear and turbid by both spleen and kidney. After discontinuing, if taken for a long period and in high doses, it will lead to yang vacuity cold and depletion of essence. I will usually prescribe the use of moxa, and formulas such as 50 percent *shèn qì wán*/kidney qi pill and 50 percent *xiǎo chái hú tāng*/minor bupleurum decoction to stabilize the body and mind.

Recreational stimulants (from cocaine and methedrine to caffeine beverages and coffee)

Stimulants tend to outthrust yang qi from the kidneys upwards to the brain, but in doing so exhaust the yang qi and *jīng* 精/essence leading to yang vacuity internal cold. In varying degrees, they speed up and lift the pulse to the exterior yang region. But over time, as the stimulants exhaust the body, the pulse will become more stagnant, choppy and soggy. Many stimulants have a hot and drying quality and consume yin qi as well.

Anti-depressants

These tend to have a stagnating, and accumulating property causing accumulation of phlegm damp. The name 'SSRI (serotonin reuptake inhibitor)' means that a normal process of reabsorption of a form of *jīng* 精/essence is allowed to facilitate accumulation of serotonin in the brain. The *nǎo* 腦/brain is associated in Chinese medicine with associated acupuncture channels, including *jué yīn* 厥陰, *shào yīn* 少陰, and *shào yáng* 少陽. So there tends to be a dulling of the *shén* 神 and *hún* 魂 specifically, the aspects of consciousness associated with the *shèn* 腎/kidneys and *gān* 肝/liver, along with a lack of discernment of the *yì* 意 (spirit associated with the spleen).

Sex hormones (specifically estrogen)

All pharmaceutically administrated hormones can be considered in Chinese medicine to be a species of 'artificial *jīng* 精'. Taking artificial *jīng* 精, due to the fact that standard hormones are fractionalized, similar to the hydrogenization of fats, they are not broken down significantly by the function of the spleen, which is to separate clear and turbid. In terms of Chinese medical characteristics, estrogen specifically tends to be cold, sweet, heavy, sinking and damp. A woman on the pill or HRT will present with a pulse that at first feels like that of a pregnant woman, slippery and *huǎn* 緩/leisurely (*huǎn mài* 緩脈/regular/leisurely pulse), which is associated with the spleen. But over time the accumulation of cold and damp in the lower burner, which inhibits fertility, also leads to cold blood stasis and the pulse becomes more and more rough and soggy to the point where it may feel suffocated as the vessels become occluded. In treatment of these patients, the Chinese medical physician can combine 50 percent *shèn qì wán*/kidney qi pill with 50 percent *guì zhī fú líng wán*/cinnamon twig and poria pill among their choices.

Antibiotics

The nature of many antibiotics is cold, bitter, dispersing, and they clear fire. This is similar in some ways to the effects of *huáng lián* 黃連/coptis, or *huáng qín* 黃芩/scutellaria. However, specifically industrial or laboratory produced antibiotics as opposed to natural ones such as penicillin are much stronger and therefore the excess bitter cold damages the spleen and stomach. In modern terms the intestinal flora and microbiome are damaged by the killing off of beneficial bacteria that aid in digestion and immunity. Many of the problems with young children in regard to the production of phlegm/damp, allergies and poor digestion can be attributed to the overuse of antibiotics. Over time, with repeated administration of antibiotics, the pulse will tend to become thinner and soggy. One of the reasons they often seem to work in largely viral conditions even though they are contraindicated is this heat-clearing aspect, but there is a large price to be paid for the indiscriminate use of antibiotics.

Vaccines

In a healthy patient, after administration many vaccines should produce some variation of an exterior reaction, such as skin rash, nausea, vomiting, joint aches, or a floating pulse. Sometimes the pulse will be rapid, sometimes *tài yáng* 太陽/floating, but a strong pulse may be produced indicating a condition *shāng hán* 傷寒/cold damage. Sometimes a floating, more relaxed pulse may indicate *zhòng fēng* 中風/wind strike.

In more extreme cases, especially in young children, a *yáng míng* 陽明/rapid flooding slippery pulse (*yáng míng* 陽明/ channel pulse) may occur. This means the body is trying to neutralize the effects of the vaccine by exteriorizing the pathogen. If the pathogen in the vaccine reaches the *shào yáng* 少陽 stage, the pulse will be wiry. The body's response to the vaccine can be supported with appropriate formulas such as *gé gēn tāng*/kudzu decoction, *guì zhī tāng* 桂枝湯/cinnamon twig decoction, or *chái hú guì zhī tāng*/bupleurum and cinnamon twig decoction, or even *bái hǔ tāng*/white tiger decoction, without neutralizing the vaccine's prophylaxis. The Chinese medical physician, of course, can apply acupuncture and/or moxibustion by treating the appropriate associated channel(s). One of the main issues with present-day vaccine programs is giving multiple vaccines, especially in a short window of time, or at an age when a child's immune response is still immature. Another factor mentioned by Chinese physicians such as Xu Da-cun is giving vaccines when a child or adult is sick. The end result if caution is not taken is confusion of the body/mind system, overwhelming the channels with confusing messages. This in turn may lead to long-term complex conditions such as allergies, and potential autoimmune complaints.

On Terminology: The Importance of Terminology and Language in Grasping Chinese Medicine

Z'ev Rosenberg, Ken Rose, and Daniel Schrier

The notion of a distributed mind is magnified by the idea that the functional mind of study is truly trans-personal. When we study and we teach, we pay attention to this trans-personal mind and ensure through nourishment and provision of insight and persistence that the community of knowledge grows and undergoes necessary refinement. All study is cultivation of the human mind, not in a limited sense, i.e., to an emanation of a solitary brain or nervous system, but in an expanded sense of developing consciousness where the mysteries of life itself remain to be discovered.

Chinese culture has always venerated ancestors within families, and cultural transmissions across time. It is no accident that the medicine of China also has been preserved and updated in this fashion. China has one of the oldest literate cultures in the world, and the vessel of transmission of Chinese medicine has always been the *jīng* 經/source text. These included philosophical texts from the early Han dynasty, including the *Dao de jing*, *Yi jing*, and *Huai nan zi*, which established the Tao, yin/yang theory, and the *wǔ xíng*/ five phases as the foundation principles on which Chinese arts, sciences, culture and medicine were to be based. The medical classics, such as the *Su wen*, *Ling shu*, and *Nan jing* continued this trend, and are the inspiration focus for this book.

In order to understand this medical transmission, the first step is to gain a working familiarity with classical Chinese language. Unlike most other languages, Chinese is essentially pictographic, especially if one traces it back to its sources in ancient character sets. It is unique in how a large amount of information (about an object or phenomenon) is embedded in a small, condensed character or character set. Through the study of essential characters such as *jīng* 經, one can gain understanding of the deeper meanings embedded in Chinese medicine and its relationship to the culture that gave birth to it. According to Sandra Hill, *jīng* 經 "suggests a transmission of information from heaven, a sacred text that gives guidance to life."[1] It has the silk thread radical (*sī* 絲) on the left, suggesting a threadlike continuity. The phonetic on the right shows streams of water flowing under the earth, describing a form of organization and regulation.

Arguments that technical mastery and knowledge are sufficient to practice Chinese medicine, that the canon is obscure and outdated, are incomplete. Such an approach to education produces technicians, treating symptoms and parts separated from the whole, who rely on biomedical diagnoses in order to treat patients. When one practices in this manner, as a large part of the profession presently does, one cannot frame the patient's sufferings within the medical tradition from which these tools arise. It becomes difficult to produce a treatment plan, diagnose, or understand within one's own medical tradition how to explain what one sees in the patient. In Chinese medicine, craft, technique and diagnostic acumen are the logical extension of study of the source material in the medical classics.

So, we can say that studying and practicing Chinese medicine is a Tao, a way of life. One "lives" Chinese medicine,

---

1   Hill 2014

through studying the seasons, circadian rhythms, methods, and self-cultivation methods revealed in the classics. This study is lifelong, it does not end with a degree, and it begins as soon as one leaves school. Without continuous study of the medical classics, one cannot develop the cognitive tools and "physician's mind" necessary to truly practice this medicine. Training the mind is concurrent with diagnostic acumen, technical skill, writing formulas, needling and applying moxibustion.

Because classical Chinese medicine (as opposed to traditional Chinese medicine or TCM) is so new in the West, study groups and communities of scholars are necessary. We have very few teachers of the medical classics, in both the acupuncture and herbal traditions, so much of this study is in our own hands. Teaching this medicine is a form of transmission through time, and there is a resonance to this teaching. In other words, truly understanding Chinese medicine is more than the memorization of facts, points, herbs, or *zàng fǔ* patterns. It is a depth of understanding, a meditation on the order of the universe through its universal principles and its resulting manifestation in nature.

This does not mean that Chinese medicine is "archaic," or closed to new advancements. Every generation has written new commentaries on medical texts, from the *Nan jing* to the *Shang han lun*, and several schools and currents have arisen to deal with new problems and issues in every dynasty and in every generation. *Lǐ lùn* 理論/principles are timeless, as timeless as the theory of conservation of energy in physics. One's applications are meant to be creative, and expressed in real-time clinical settings.

It is those who take up the challenges of this study and practice who will not only preserve Chinese medicine for future generations, but allow it to advance and grow in the fertile soil of the West.

Resources for Learning Medical Chinese Language

Software and applications

Wenlin—http://wenlin.com (for MacOS and Windows)

A comprehensive portable tool for students and scholars. Includes multiple dictionaries for learning, reading, and writing Chinese language. With a comprehensive character dictionary, it has over 73,000 characters, with 200,000 Chinese words and phrases. Gives access to expandable Chinese dictionaries, a full-featured text editor, and a unique "flashcard" system.

Pleco Chinese Dictionary—www.pleco.com (for Apple iOS devices and Android devices)

An integrated dictionary (Oxford, Longman, FLTRP (Foreign Language Teaching and Research Press), Wiseman and Ye's *A Practical Dictionary of Chinese Medicine*, Kroll's *A Student's Dictionary of Classical and Medieval Chinese*, as well as many others), document reader (which supports TXT/EPUB/DOC/PDF files and web pages on iOS, TXT/PDF files on Android), flashcards, full-screen handwriting input and optical character recognizer (OCR) to look up unknown Chinese words "live" or from still image photos using your device's camera.

Outlier Dictionary of Chinese Characters—
www.outlier-linguistics.com/#3editions
(Pleco add-on for MacOS and Windows)

A wonderful add-on to Pleco, which comes in three editions. *The Mini Edition* contains 2000 characters, in Simplified and Traditional, with full, detailed entries for all semantic components, and has 300+ entries, including the ancient forms. *The Essential Edition* contains the same as *The Mini Edition* but with 2000 more characters. There is a bilingual function with Chinese plus either English or German, and a System Tab, to see the connections between characters. *The Expert Edition* contains the same as *The Essential Edition* and includes the ancient forms for all characters. There is detailed historical and etymological information for all the characters. (Note: *The Essential Edition* and *The Expert Edition* are only available for pre-order currently.)

Books

Practical Dictionary of Chinese Medicine
by Nigel Wiseman and Feng Ye

Provides a wealth of useful information beyond the definition of terms. There are cross-references that lead the reader from familiar to less familiar concepts, and there is a standard for the use of words that properly links English terminology to the Chinese. It defines each term clearly and concisely, giving the original Chinese term and its tone-marked Pinyin transcription. It provides synonyms and abbreviations where necessary, and offers etymologies for key terms.

A Student's Dictionary of Classical and Medieval Chinese by Paul Kroll

A Chinese to English reference work, this is excellent for texts dating from the Warring States (475–221 BC) through the Tang dynasty (618–906 CE). Comprises over 8,000 characters, and is arranged alphabetically by Pinyin, with an index by radical and stroke-count.

Dictionary of the Ben can gang mu, Volume 1: Chinese Historical Illness Terminology
by Zhang Zhibin and Paul Unschuld

Analyzes the meaning of 4500 historical illness terms from 1500 years of Chinese medical observation and theorization. Many of the terms employed often fail to overlap with modern biomedical terminology. Though the text includes an extensive list of illness terminology, it does not include the entirety of the pre-modern illness terms. In addition, because this is a pharmaceutical text, many of the terms used are more for a pharmaceutical-based treatment.

Chinese Medical Chinese: Grammar and Vocabulary by Nigel Wiseman and Feng Ye

Describes the basic features of literary Chinese medical language and its relationship to both the classical language and the modern language. Explaining many grammatical constructions commonly encountered in Chinese medical texts, this describes how Chinese medical terms are composed, as well as presenting vocabulary and terminology of Chinese medicine and its component characters. The book covers basic theories, four examinations, diseases, patho-mechanisms and disease patterns, principles and methods of treatment, pharmaceutics, and acupuncture. It includes etymologies of terms, gives component characters in simplified and complex form, and explains term translations for 1027 characters and 2555 compound terms.

Learn to Read Chinese, Volumes I and II by Paul Unschuld

These two volumes teach the language of contemporary Chinese technical literature. The texts chosen are from the introduction to Chinese medicine written by Qin Bowei, one of the founders of TCM and a medical writer known for his clear, precise, and detailed clinical expression. The first volume teaches vocabulary, with exercises for the readers to transliterate, then translate a passage based on the simplified character vocabulary provided with each passage and its preceding passages. The second volume teaches analysis of Chinese texts through the principles of natural language development. By showing how to identify the basic statement in a sentence and the adjunct statements that complete its meaning, just as children learn to read their native language, it gives the reader access to Chinese texts as quickly as possible. When the course is completed, users are working with typical modern Chinese medical sources.

Chinese Life Sciences: Introductory Readings in Classical Chinese Medicine by Paul Unschuld

A selection of 60 texts compiled and translated from 33 classics including the *Huang di nei jing, Yi xue, Nan jing, Shi ji, San yin lun, Shang han lun, Ben cao gan mu,* and *Pi wei lun.* Presented in ten lessons each with vocabulary and translations.

Online databases

Chinese Text Project—http://ctext.org

An online open-access digital library that makes pre-modern Chinese texts available to readers and researchers all around the world. The site makes use of the digital medium to explore new ways of interacting with these texts that are not possible in print. With over 30,000 titles and more than five billion characters, the Chinese Text Project is also the largest database of pre-modern Chinese texts.

Online dictionaries

MDBG English to Chinese Dictionary—www.mdbg.net/chinese/dictionary (also available for MacOS and Window)

A free online English to Chinese/Chinese to English dictionary, this offers various tools such as flashcards, quizzes, text annotation, and Chinese text input.

ChineseEtymology—http://chineseetymology.org

Created by Richard Sears, this website is dedicated to providing information on the various early forms of Chinese characters, in an easily searchable format, by typing or pasting in the Chinese character. It provides a basic English meaning in the sidebar.

Online Chinese Medical Dictionary—www.paradigm-pubs.com/book/export/html/380

Containing over 30,000 terms, this is one of the largest Chinese to English/English to Chinese listings of Chinese medical terms. It uses the *Practical Dictionary of Chinese Medicine*, by Wiseman and Feng (Paradigm Publications) as the source for the English terminology is that represented.

Different Pulse Maps from Classical Texts and Physician's Schools

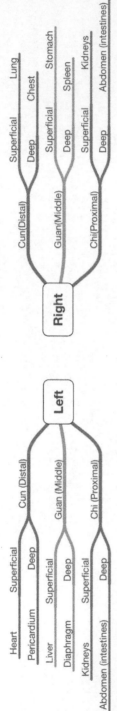

Figure Appendix 4.1: Nei jing Su wen pulse model

Figure Appendix 4.2: Chen Yan pulse model

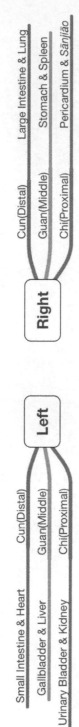

Figure Appendix 4.3: Liu Wan-su pulse model

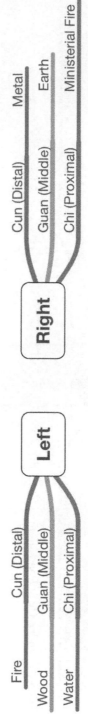

Figure Appendix 4.4: Hua Shou pulse model

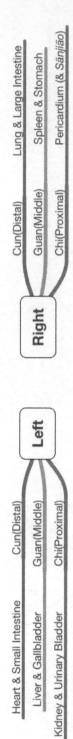

Figure Appendix 4.5: Li Dong-yuan pulse model

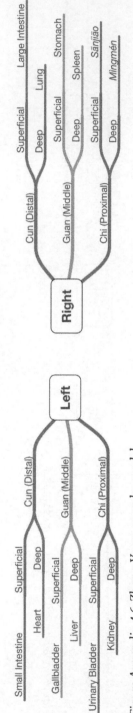

Figure Appendix 4.6: Zhang Yuan-su pulse model

Abdominal Algorithms: Qualities of Palpation

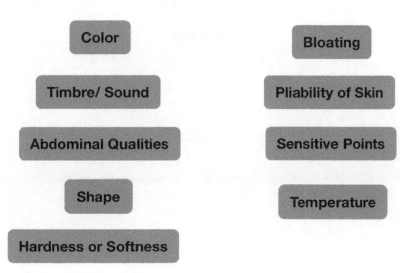

Figure Appendix 5.1: Abdominal algorithms

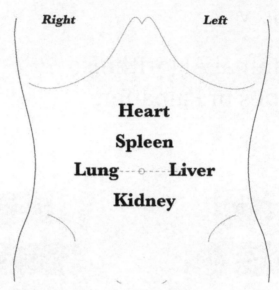

Figure Appendix 5.2: Nan jing 16 Abdominal map

Nan jing 18 Pulse Model

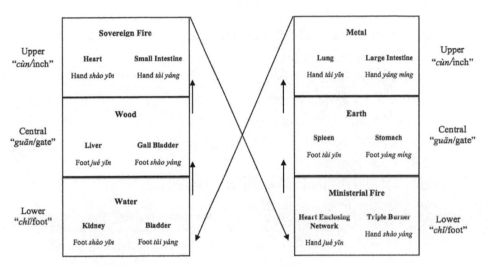

Figure Appendix 6.1: Nan jing 18 pulse model

Glossary of Terms

bā gāng biàn zhèng 八綱辨證 Eight principle pattern identification

biàn 變 Transformation, to change

biàn zhèng 辨證 Pattern identification

biāo běn 標本 Root and branch

bié mài 別脈 Divergent vessels

bìng yīn 病因 Disease origin or etiology; cause of disease

bǔ 補 Supplementation

cùn kǒu 寸口 Inch opening; location of the radial pulse

cùn 寸 Inch, guān 關 Gate (bar)/ and chǐ 尺 Foot (cubit)

dà qì 大氣 Great qi/air qi (the qi of the environment, air…the important qi. Refers here to the qi of the universe that enters the body though inhalation)

dà yī 大醫 (great physician) *shàng gōng* 上工 (superior physician) The highest level of doctors as defined in the classic medical texts such as the *Huáng dì nèi jīng* (*Sù wèn* and *Líng shū*), *Nán jīng*, and *Jīn guì yào lü*

dào 道 The Way; the movement of life

dào dì yào cái 道地藥材 Genuine/authentic medicinal

dì 地 Earth

dòng qì 動氣 Stirring qi

duì yào 對藥 Herbal pairing—combination of the selecting two herbs that become more beneficial than the individual herb

fǔ 腑 Bowels

gǎn yìng 感應 Resonance

gōng xié 攻邪 Attacking (disease) evils

gōu 鉤 Hook

gǔ qì 穀氣 Food/grain qi, this is a reference to yang qi, derived from the consumption of food

hàn 汗 Sweating

hé 和 Harmonization

hé bìng 合病 Combination diseases of multiple channels

huà 化 To change into; to transform

huǎn 緩 Construed as a normal pulse, it is even and moderate, and is the sign of the presence of stomach qi; construed as a pathological pulse, it is forceless, and is mostly seen in dampness patterns and spleen-stomach vacuity

huì xué 會穴 Meeting point

hún 魂 Spirit associated with the liver

jīn yè biàn zhèng 津液辨證 Fluids pattern differentiation

jīng 精 Essence; that which is responsible for growth, development and reproduction, and determines the strength of the constitution

jīng 經 Channel; classical text

jīng luò 經絡 Channels and network (connecting) vessels.

jīng luò biàn zhèng 經絡辨證 Channel and network vessel pattern differentiation

jīng mài 經脈 Channel/vessel system

jīng qì 精氣 Essential qi; any essential element of the body (blood, qi, fluid, essence); specifically, the acquired essence and the essence stored by the viscera and indissociable from the essential qi that is stored by the kidney and used in reproduction

jiǔ ruò 灸焫 To cauterize (moxibustion)

jiǔ zhēn 九針 Nine needles (of acupuncture)

jūn huǒ 君火 Sovereign fire

kè 尅 Control; restrain (five-phase cycle)

kè qì 客氣 Guest qi

láo sǔn 勞損 Vacuity taxation; taxation detriment

liù jīng biàn zhèng 六經辨證 Six channel pattern differentiation

luò mài 絡脈 Network vessels

mài xiàng 脈象 Pulse imagery

mài zhěn 脈診 Pulse examination

máo 毛 Hair-like

mìng mén 命門 Life gate

mìng mén huǒ 命門火 Life gate fire

nèi shāng 內傷 Internal damage; internal injury

nǎo 腦 Brain

nì 逆 To oppose, go against, to flow counter to the normal direction

páo zhì 炮製 Processing of medicinals

páng guāng 膀胱 Bladder channel

qì 氣 That which animates, transforms and maintains all life; often translated as energy or vital energy. A fundamental concept in Chinese medicine

qì huà 氣化 Qi transformation; the movement, mutation, and conversion of qi

qì xuè biàn zhèng 氣血辨證 Qi/blood pattern differentiation

qīng 清 Clear, clearing

qīng 清 *dàn* 淡 'Clear-bland'

qīng qì 氣 Clear qi

rén 人 Humanity; man

rú yī 儒醫 Scholar-physician. A concept developed during the 12th century Song dynasty through the encouragement of the emperor where the practice of medicine was elevated to a higher social status. These scholar-physicians studied and had an understanding of the classical texts such as the *Sù wèn*, *Líng shū*, and *Nán jīng* to understand channel/connecting vessel theory, the *Shāng hán zá bìng lùn* to diagnose progressions of disease parts and practice internal medicine

sān jiāo 三焦 Three burners/three heaters; one of the six fu

sān jiāo biàn zhèng 三焦辨證 Three-burner pattern differentiation

sǎn mài 散脈 Scattered pulse, dissipated pulse

sè 澀 Choppy, rough,

shāng hán 傷寒 Cold damage

shén 神 Spirit; consciousness

shēng 生 Generating cycle

shí 石 Stone-like

shùn 順 Obey, submit to, go along with

si da jia 四大家 Four great physicians (Li Wan-su, Zhang Zi-he, Li Dong-yuan, and Zhu Dan-xi) *sì fēn biàn zhèng* 四分辨證 Four-aspect pattern differentiation

tiān 天 Heaven

tù 吐 Ejection (vomiting)

wài gǎn 外感 External contractions

wèi qì 衛氣 Defense qi; the superficially protective aspect of the circulation of qi that is within the channels and defends the body from outside invasion

wēn 溫 Warming

wǔ shū xué 五输穴 Five transport points

wǔ xíng biàn zhèng 五行辨證 Five-phase pattern differentiation

wǔ xíng xué shuō 五行學說 Five-phase theory

wǔ yùn liù qì 五運六氣 Five periods and six qi; chronobiology theory

wǔ zàng 五臟 Five viscera (heart/*xīn* 心, liver/*gān* 肝, spleen/*pí* 脾, lungs/*fèi* 肺 and kidneys/*shèn* 腎)

xiàn 線 Tense/wiry, string-like

xiāo 消 Dispersing

xiàng 象 Image; reflection; likeness; portrait, picture; statue

xiàng huǒ 相火 Ministerial fire

xiè 瀉 Draining

xié qì 邪氣 Evil qi; unhealthy influences that cause disease; pathogenic invasive agent which usually enters the body from the outside

xīn zhǔ 心主 Heart governor

xué 穴 Hole, acupuncture point

yào cǎo 藥草 Medicinal herb

yǎng shēng 養生 Nourishing life, a term that covers the health preservation practices that have been an important part of health care since early times, and which remain important today. These include physical exercises, diet, lifestyle regulation, and sexual practices

yì 意 Spirit associated with the spleen

yī 醫 Medicine, doctor, to cure, to treat

yī xué 醫學 Medicine; medical science; study of medicine

yīn yáng 陰陽 The two fundamental aspects of the universe; the shady and sunny side of the mountain,

yíng qì 營氣 Construction, provisioning

yù hòu 預後 Prognosis

yuán qì 原氣 Source qi; the basic form of qi in the body, which is made up of a combination of three other forms of qi: the essential qi of the kidney; qi of grain and water, derived through the transformative function of the spleen; and air (great qi), drawn in through the lung

yuán wù bǐ lèi 援物比類 Grasping the cause, making an analogy

zàng 臟 Viscera; viscus, any of the five viscera (lung, kidney, liver, heart, and spleen)

zàng fǔ biàn zhèng 臟腑辨證 Bowel and visceral pattern differentiation; organ pattern differentiation

zàng qì 臟氣 Visceral qi

zàng xiàng 臟象 Visceral manifestation

zàng qì xué 臟器學 Visceral form theory

zhěn duàn 診斷 To diagnose; diagnosis

zhèng cháng mài 正常脈 Normal pulse

zhèng qì 正氣 Right qi; correct qi; true qi; upright qi

zhōng 中 Center, (position associated with *dì* 地/earth); central, middle

zhòng fēng 中風 Wind strike

zhōng jiāo 中焦 Central burner (of the spleen and stomach)

zhuó qì 濁氣 Turbid qi

zhì 志 Will (the spirit of the kidneys), intention, aspiration,

zhǔ qì 主氣 Host qi; governing qi

Classical Texts

Authors	Pinyin title	English Title	Date
Anonymous	**Zhōu yì** 周易 (**Yì jīng** 易經)	Changes of the Zhou Dynasty (Classic of Changes)	c.-1000 to -50
Anonymous	**Huáng dì nèi jīng sù wèn** 黃帝內經素問	Yellow Emperor's Internal Classic— Plain Question	c.-100
Anonymous	**Huáng dì nèi jīng líng shū** 黃帝內經靈樞	Yellow Emperor's Internal Classic— The Divine Pivot	c.-100
Anonymous	**Nán jīng** 難經	The Classic of Difficulties	c.-100
Anonymous	**Shén nóng běn cǎo jīng** 神農本草經	Shen Nong's Materia Medica	c.+100
Zhāng Zhòng Jǐng	**Shāng hán zá bìng lùn** (**Shāng hán lùn** & **Jīn guì yào lüè**) 傷寒雜病論(傷寒論&金匱要略)	Essays on Cold Attack and Miscellaneous Disease/ Treatise on Cold Damage and Complex Diseases	c.+220
Wáng Shū Hē	**Mài jīng** 脈經	Pulse Classic	c.310

Authors	Pinyin title	English Title	Date
Huáng Fǔ Mì	Jiǎ yǐ jīng 甲乙經 (Zhēn jiǔ jiǎ yǐ jīng 針灸甲乙經)	Systematic Classic of Acumoxa	259
Sūn Sī Miǎo	Qiān jīn yào fāng 千金要方	The Essential Prescriptions Worth a Thousand in Gold	652
Lǐ Dōng Yuán (Lǐ Gǎo)	Pí wèi lùn 脾胃論	Treatise on the Spleen and Stomach	1249
Lǐ Shí Zhēn	Bīn hú mài xué 瀕湖脈學	Lakeside Pulse Classic	1564
Lǐ Shí Zhēn	Běn cǎo gāng mù 本草綱目	Compendium of Medical Herbs	1596
Yáng Jì Zhōu	Zhēn jiǔ dà chéng 針灸大成	Great Compendium of Acumoxa	1601
Wú Qiān	Yī zōng jīn jiàn 醫宗金鑑	The Golden Mirror of Medicine	1742
Wú Táng	Wēn bìng tiáo bian 溫病條辨	Systematized Identification of Warm Diseases	1798
Zhèng Qīn Ān	Yī lǐ zhēn chuán 醫理真傳	Medical Principles' True Transmission	1869

References

Bernard, C., Greene, H.C., Henderson, L.J. and Cohen, I. B. (2013) *An Introduction to the Study of Experimental Medicine*. New York: Dover Publications.

Dharmasiri, G. (1997) *The Nature of Medicine: A Critique of the Myth of Medicine*. Kandy, Sri Lanka: Gunapala Dharmasiri.

Foucault, M. (2003) *The Birth of the Clinic: An Archaeology of Medical Perception*. London: Routledge.

Hill, S. (2014) *Chinese Medicine from the Classics: A Beginner's Guide*. London: Monkey Press.

Hillis, D. (2010) *Edge Master Class 2010: W. Daniel Hillis on "Cancering."* Retrieved from www.edge.org/event/edge-master-class-2010-w-daniel-hillis-on-cancering.

Hsu, E. (2008) "A hybrid body technique: Does the pulse diagnostic cun guan chi method have Chinese Tibetan origins?" *Gesnerus, 65*, 5–29.

Langford, J.M. (1999) "Medical mimesis: healing signs of a cosmopolitan 'quack'." *American Ethnologist, 26*(1), 24–46.

Li, G. and Flaws, B. (2004) *Li Dong-yuan's Treatise on the Spleen and Stomach: A Translation of the Pi Wei Lun*. Boulder, CO: Blue Poppy.

Lightman, A. (2004) *Einstein's Dreams*. New York, NY: Vintage.

Mahdi, M. (2001) *Alfarabi: Philosophy of Plato and Aristotle*. Ithaca, NY: Cornell University Press.

Manaka, Y., Itaya, K. and Birch, S. (1995) *Chasing the Dragon's Tail: The Theory and Practice of Acupuncture in the Work of Yoshio Manaka*. Brookline, MA: Paradigm Publications.

Qu, L. and Garvey, M. (2008) "Chinese medicine and the yi jing's epistemic methodology." *Australian Journal of Acupuncture and Chinese Medicine, 3*(1), 17–23. Retrieved from www.biroco.com/yijing/Yijing_and_chinese_medicine.pdf.

Rossi, E. (2007) *Shen: Psycho-Emotional Aspects of Chinese Medicine*. Edinburgh: Churchill Livingstone Elsevier.

Scheid, V. (2007) *Currents of Tradition 1626–2006.* Seattle, WA: Eastland Press.

Scheid, V. (2009) "The Mangle of Practice and the Practice of Chinese Medicine: A Case Study from 19th Century China." In A. Pickering and K. Guzik (eds) *The Mangle in Practice: Science, Society, and Becoming* (pp.110–128). Durham, NC: Duke University Press.

Shubin, N. (2013, January 26) *January is the Cruelest Month.* Retrieved from www.nytimes.com/2013/01/27/opinion/sunday/for-sleep-january-is-the-cruelest-month.html?_r=0.

Sivin, N. (1987) "On the Limits of Empirical Knowledge in the Traditional Chinese Sciences." In J.T. Fraser, F.C. Haber and N.M. Lawrence (eds) *Time, Science and Society in China and the West* (pp.151–169). London: University of Massachusetts Press/Eurospan.

Sun, S. (2012) *Qianjinfang Ethics: Volume One, Chapter Two: On the Sublime Sincerity of the Eminent Physician* (S. Wilms trans.). Retrieved from www.happygoatproductions.com/qianjinfang-ethics.

Unschuld, P. (2003) "The Yellow Emperor's Classics: The Messages of the Huang Di Nei Jing Su Wen and the Nan Jing." Lecture presented at Pacific Symposium 11 November 2003 in California, San Diego.

Unschuld, P. (2016) *Huang Di Nei Jing Ling Shu: The Ancient Classic on Needle Therapy: The Complete Chinese Text with an Annotated English Translation.* Oakland, CA: University of California Press.

Unschuld, P. (2016) *Nan Jing: The Classic of Difficult Issues.* Berkeley, CA: University of California Press.

Unschuld, P. and Tessenow, H. (2011) *Huang Di Nei Jing Su Wen: An Annotated Translation of Huang Di's Inner Classic—Basic Questions, 2 Volumes.* Berkeley, CA: University of California Press.

Velasquez-Manoff, M. (2013) *An Epidemic of Absence: A New Way of Understanding Allergies and Autoimmune Diseases.* New York, NY: Scribner.

Welden, J. (2015) *To Bring Order Out of Chaos: Literati Medicine of the Jin Dynasty (1115-1234)* (Doctoral dissertation, University of Hawaii Manoa). (UMI No. 3717248).

Wiseman, N., and Ye, F. (1998) *Practical Dictionary of Chinese Medicine.* Taos, NM: Paradigm Press.

Zhang, X. (2009) *On the Relationship Between Medicine and Philosophy.* Classical Chinese Medicine: translation and introduction (H. Fruehuaf trans.). Retrieved from https://classicalchinesemedicine.org/wp-content/uploads/2016/03/fruehauf_zhangxichun-relationshipENG.pdf.

Index